Neuroscience

Guest Editor

ANNE ALEXANDROV, PhD, RN, CCRN, FAAN

CRITICAL CARE NURSING CLINICS OF NORTH AMERICA

www.ccnursing.theclinics.com

Consulting Editor
JANET FOSTER, PhD, RN, CNS

December 2009 • Volume 21 • Number 4

SAUNDERS an imprint of ELSEVIER, Inc.

W.B. SAUNDERS COMPANY
A Division of Elsevier Inc.

Elsevier Inc., 1600 John F. Kennedy Blvd., Suite 1800, Philadelphia, PA 19103-2899

http://www.theclinics.com

CRITICAL CARE NURSING CLINICS OF NORTH AMERICA Volume 21, Number 4
December 2009 ISSN 0899-5885, ISBN-13: 978-1-4377-1205-6, ISBN-10: 1-4377-1205-3

Editor: Katie Hartner
Developmental Editor: Donald Mumford

Critical Care Nursing Clinics of North America (ISSN 0899-5885) is published quarterly by Elsevier Inc., 360 Park Avenue South, New York, NY 10010-1710. Months of issue are March, June, September, and December. Business and Editorial Offices: 1600 John F. Kennedy Blvd., Suite 1800, Philadelphia, PA 19103-2899. Periodicals postage paid at New York, NY and additional mailing offices. Subscription prices are $130.00 per year for US individuals, $233.00 per year for US institutions, $68.00 per year for US students and residents, $167.00 per year for Canadian individuals, $292.00 per year for Canadian institutions, $191.00 per year for international individuals, $292.00 per year for international institutions and $99.00 per year for Canadian and foreign students/residents. To receive student/resident rate, orders must be accompanied by name of affiliated institution, data of term, and the *signature* of program/residency coordinator on institution letterhead. Orders will be billed at individual rate until proof of status is received. Foreign air speed delivery is included in all *Clinics* subscription prices. All prices are subject to change without notice. **POSTMASTER:** Send address changes to *Critical Care Nursing Clinics of North America*, Elsevier Health Sciences Division, Subscription Customer Service, 3251 Riverport Lane, Maryland Heights, MO 63043. **Customer Service: 1-800-654-2452 (US and Canada); 314-447-8871 (outside US and Canada). Fax: 314-447-8029. E-mail: JournalsCustomerService-usa@elsevier.com (for print support) and JournalsOnlineSupport-usa@elsevier.com (for online support).**

Reprints. For copies of 100 or more of articles in this publication, please contact the Commercial Reprints Department, Elsevier Inc., 360 Park Avenue South, New York, New York, 10010-1710; Tel.: (212) 633-3813, Fax: (212) 462-1935, and E-mail: reprints@elsevier.com.

Critical Care Nursing Clinics of North America is covered in *MEDLINE/PubMed (Index Medicus), International Nursing Index, Nursing Citation Index, Cumulative Index to Nursing and Allied Health Literature,* and *RNdex Top 100.*

Printed in the United States of America.

Contributors

GUEST EDITOR

ANNE W. WOJNER ALEXANDROV, PhD, RN, CCRN, FAAN
Professor, School of Nursing; Professor, School of Medicine; and Comprehensive
Stroke Center; Program Director, NET SMART (Neurovascular Education and Training
in Stroke Management and Acute Reperfusion Therapy), University of Alabama
at Birmingham, Birmingham, Alabama

AUTHORS

ANNE W. WOJNER ALEXANDROV, PhD, RN, CCRN, FAAN
Professor, School of Nursing; Professor, School of Medicine; and Comprehensive Stroke
Center; Program Director, NET SMART (Neurovascular Education and Training in Stroke
Management and Acute Reperfusion Therapy), University of Alabama at Birmingham,
Birmingham, Alabama

TRACEY ANDERSON, MSN, CNRN, FNP-BC
Neurocritical Care and Neurosurgery Nurse Practitioner, University of Colorado Hospital,
Aurora, Colorado; Instructor, Department of Neurosurgery, University of Colorado, School
of Medicine, University of Colorado Denver, Aurora, Colorado

SHARON BIBY, MSN, RN, ANP
Nurse Practitioner and Stroke Center Director, Moses Cone Health System, Greensboro,
North Carolina

MARY BRETHOUR, MSN, RN, ACNP
Neurovascular Nurse Practitioner, University of Alabama at Birmingham, Comprehensive
Stroke Center, Birmingham, Alabama

FERN CUDLIP, MSN, RN, ANP
Stroke Program Clinical Director, Eden Medical Center, Castro Valley, California

CINDY J. FULLER, PhD
Clinical Assistant Professor, Department of Cardiovascular Scientific Development,
University of Washington School of Nursing, Swedish Medical Center, Seattle,
Washington

DIANE HANDLER, MSN, RN, CNS
Stroke Coordinator, Mercy Medical Center, Cedar Rapids, Iowa

JILL T. JESURUM, PhD, ARNP, FAHA
Research Assistant Professor, Department of Cardiovascular Scientific Development,
University of Washington School of Nursing, Swedish Medical Center, Seattle,
Washington

TERRI-ELLEN KIERNAN, MSN, RN, ANP
Nurse Practitioner, Cerebrovascular Neurology, Mayo Clinic, Phoenix, Arizona

LORETTA T. LEE, RN, MSN, CRNP,
Adult/Gerontology Nurse Practitioner Program, Department of Adult/Acute Health, Chronic Care and Foundations; University of Alabama School of Nursing, Birmingham, Alabama

DAWN MEYER, MSN, FNP, RN, PhD(c)
Sharp Memorial Hospital, Ortho/Neuro Services, San Diego, California

DANA REINER, MSN, RN, ANP
Neurovascular Nurse Practitioner, St Joseph's Regional Medical Center, Paterson, New Jersey

ROBIN L. SAIKI, MSN, RN, ACNP
Instructor, Department of Neurosurgery, University of Colorado Health Sciences Center, Aurora, Colorado

DANA A. STRADLING, RN, BSN, CNRN
Stroke Program Manager, UC Irvine, Orange, California

VICTORIA SWATZELL, MSN, RN, ANP
Neurovascular Nurse Practitioner Scottsdale Healthcare Osborn, Scottsdale, Arizona

SUSAN TOCCO, MSN, RN, CNS
Neurovascular Clinical Nurse Specialist, Orlando Regional Medical Center, Orlando, Florida

THERESA M. WADAS, PhD(c), RN, FNP-BC, ACNP-BC, CCRN
Clinical Faculty, Adult Acute Nurse Practitioner Program, School of Nursing, University of Alabama at Birmingham, Birmingham, Alabama; PhD Candidate, Nursing, Injury Mechanisms, College of Nursing, University of Arizona, Tucson, Arizona

JOANNA YANG, MSN, RN, ANP
Nurse Practitioner/Clinical Nurse Specialist and Stroke Program Coordinator, Loma Linda University Medical Center, Loma Linda, California

SUSAN YEAGER, MS, RN, CCRN, ACNP
Trauma/Acute and Emergency Surgery, Nurse Practitioner, The Ohio State University Medical Center, Columbus, Ohio

Contents

> The *Neurovascular Education and Training in Stroke Management and
> Acute Reperfusion Therapy* (NET SMART) program for advanced practice
> nursing (APN) offers a first-of-its-kind, academic, postgraduate, fellowship
> program for APNs that is modeled after physician academic fellowship
> programs but supported by a flexible Internet-based platform. This article
> details the rationale, methods, and preliminary results of the NET SMART
> APN experience, which serves as a unique template for the development
> of academic postgraduate nursing fellowship programs across a variety
> of specialty practices.

> Management of acute ischemic stroke patients is organized around sev-
> eral priorities aimed at ensuring optimal patient outcomes, the first of
> which is reperfusion therapy, followed by determination of pathogenic
> mechanism by provision of a comprehensive workup to determine proba-
> ble cause of the ischemic stroke or transient ischemic attack, for the
> purpose of providing appropriate prophylaxis for subsequent events.
> Provision of secondary prevention measures along with therapies that pre-
> vent complications associated with neurologic disability, and evaluation
> for the most appropriate level of rehabilitation services are the final prior-
> ities during acute hospitalization. This article provides an overview of
> reperfusion therapies and emerging hemodynamic treatments for hyper-
> acute ischemic strokes. Gaps in the scientific evidence that are driving
> current blood flow augmentation research are identified.

> Migraine is a prominent cause of recurrent pain, affecting 12% of the pop-
> ulation. In several case series, approximately 50% of migraineurs with aura
> were found to have patent foramen ovale (PFO). The pathophysiological
> mechanism is speculated to be passage of microemboli and vasoactive
> chemicals through the PFO, thereby evading pulmonary filtration and trig-
> gering migraine symptoms. This article presents the results of retrospec-
> tive and prospective research studies documenting the effects of PFO
> closure on migraine symptoms and presents emerging theories on

possible pathologic mechanisms that may partially explain the increased risk of ischemic stroke in the migraine population. Finally, evidence-based recommendations are presented for health care providers for managing patients who have migraine and PFO.

Despite newer neuroimaging techniques, timely and accurate diagnosis of acute stroke remains a significant challenge. The ability to identify stroke patients rapidly using a biologic biomarker would be highly beneficial. Inflammation following stroke is one physiologic mechanism that has been studied extensively in biomarker research. Several emerging inflammatory biomarkers have been identified and may be useful to diagnosis stroke, to predict the evolution of stroke, and to predict hemorrhagic transformation, particularly with the administration of thrombolytic therapy. Many challenges must be overcome before application to clinical practice can be recommended. Nevertheless, emerging inflammatory biomarkers demonstrate considerable promise, particularly as part of a multiple biomarker strategy, and significant improvement in stroke diagnosis, clinical management, and outcomes may be realized.

Hyperglycemia is a common problem in the diabetic patient after an acute stroke. Maintaining therapeutic blood glucose levels in diabetics during extreme physiologic stress can present extreme challenges. Reasonably tight, yet therapeutic, control of glycemia in the diabetic stroke patient must be a priority. This article evaluates strategies for lowering glycemia to improve neurologic outcome in acute stroke patients. It reviews the literature of the epidemiology, describes the pathophysiologic process, discusses the debate over the glycemic target goal, and gives algorithms for glucose control methods for acute care.

This article reviews the current use of antiplatelet medications in secondary stroke prevention and in acute stroke treatment. Antiplatelet medications prevent emboli and thrombus formation to avert further vascular occlusion and ischemia. Aspirin, clopidogrel (Plavix), and extended release aspirin/dipyridamole (Aggrenox) represent the mainstay of secondary prevention of ischemic and transient ischemic stroke. Although antiplatelet medications prevent platelet aggregation by different mechanisms, the end result is a significantly decreased risk of secondary stroke, myocardial infarction, and death. Increasingly, the literature reflects hypotheses about the potential utility of aspirin and clopidogrel antiplatelet therapy as a preventative measure in patients at risk of stroke and as an approach to treat embolic ischemic stroke in the acute phase once it has occurred.

Preface

The neurosciences comprise complex medical conditions, requiring not only a sound understanding of the most challenging human physiologic concepts but also provision of significantly vigilant nursing care. For these reasons, the neurosciences are regularly ranked among the most undesirable practice specialties for nurses. Making neuroscience care even less desirable for many years was the lack of any definitive treatments to reduce disability or death. But in 1995 this changed with the release of the National Institute of Neurological Disorders and Stroke tissue-type plasminogen activator (tPA) study, which showed the efficacy of tPA for treatment of acute ischemic stroke.

Approval of tPA by the US Food and Drug Administration in 1996 catapulted the neurosciences, in particular stroke care, to a position commanding attention in the health care community. Suddenly, terms, such as Decade of the Brain, stood for real change in neuroscience practice paradigms, and a significant degree of experimentation dealing with reperfusion methods, control of mechanisms associated with secondary brain injury, and other important advancements emerged.

Today, the neurosciences, in particular acute stroke care, have a commanding presence in the health care arena. Not only is there Joint Commission stroke center certification to contend with but also the Centers for Medicare & Medicaid Services stroke quality indicators, which take effect in October 2009. With the neurosciences finally front and center in acute care, nurses must commit to expanding their knowledge not only of difficult physiologic concepts but also of systems requirements tied to optimal patient and hospital outcomes.

This issue provides an overview of the newest treatments and emerging science guiding acute neuroscience care. The clinical practice topics selected include the hyperacute management of ischemic stroke, subarachnoid hemorrhage, traumatic brain injury, antiplatelet secondary stroke prevention methods, patent foramen ovale and migraine, glucose control in neuroscience patients, and emerging inflammatory biomarkers in acute stroke. Additionally, two articles present important methods to enhance advance practice nurses' contribution to neuroscience patients, including description of the first academic postgraduate fellowship for advance practice nurses in neurovascular practice.

Acute neuroscience nurses are well positioned to drive health care quality in their local practice sites. Given the complexity of the neurosciences and the growing need for rapid delivery of challenging treatments, each of us should strive to recruit future and current colleagues into this exciting, yet underserved, practice area. Although this issue provides a glimpse of current and evolving disease mechanisms and management, the rapidity with which neuroscience care is changing requires

Crit Care Nurs Clin N Am 21 (2009) ix–x
doi:10.1016/j.ccell.2009.09.003
0899-5885/09/$ – see front matter

a constant eye on the literature. My fellow authors and I hope that this issue will further our readers' neuroscience mastery and stimulate a philosophy of clinical inquiry that is tied to practice improvement for this challenging population of patients.

Anne W. Wojner Alexandrov, PhD, RN, CCRN, FAAN
School of Nursing
School of Medicine
Comprehensive Stroke Center
NET SMART (Neurovascular Education and
Training in Stroke Management and Acute Reperfusion Therapy)
University of Alabama at Birmingham
1813 6th Avenue South
UAB Hospital Russel Wing, Suite 226
Birmingham, AL 35429, USA

E-mail address:
annealex@uab.edu; http://www.netsmart-stroke.com

Postgraduate Fellowship Education and Training for Nurses: The NET SMART Experience

Anne W. Wojner Alexandrov, PhD, RN, CCRN, FAAN[a,*],
Mary Brethour, MSN, RN, ACNP[a], Fern Cudlip, MSN, RN, ANP[b],
Victoria Swatzell, MSN, RN, ANP[c], Sharon Biby, MSN, RN, ANP[d],
Dana Reiner, MSN, RN, ANP[e], Terri-Ellen Kiernan, MSN, RN, ANP[f],
Diane Handler, MSN, RN, CNS[g], Susan Tocco, MSN, RN, CNS[h],
Joanna Yang, MSN, RN, ANP[i]

KEYWORDS

- NET SMART • Post-graduate nurse fellowship programs
- Advanced practice nursing • Neurovascular advanced practice
- Stroke

Graduate nursing education prepares nurses for entry into advanced practice nursing (APN) roles, such as nurse anesthetist, nurse midwife, clinical nurse specialist (CNS), and nurse practitioner (NP). Knowledge and skills acquired through formal graduate education provide a foundation for entry into these new roles yet are insufficient to support the significant degree of specialization often expected within the practice sector. To further development and specialization in practice after graduation, nurses have relied on a variety of strategies, including conference attendance, reading professional publications, and nonstandardized mentoring by physician specialists

[a] University of Alabama at Birmingham, Comprehensive Stroke Center, 1813 6th Avenue South, UAB Hospital Russell Wing, Suite 226, Birmingham, AL 35249, USA
[b] Eden Medical Center, Castro Valley, CA, USA
[c] Scottsdale Healthcare Osborn, Scottsdale, AZ, USA
[d] Moses Cone Health System, Greensboro, NC, USA
[e] St Joseph's Regional Medical Center, Paterson, NJ, USA
[f] Cerebrovascular Neurology, Mayo Clinic, Phoenix, AZ, USA
[g] Mercy Medical Center, Cedar Rapids, IA, USA
[h] Orlando Regional Medical Center, Orlando, FL, USA
[i] Loma Linda University Medical Center, Loma Linda, CA, USA
* Corresponding author. University of Alabama at Birmingham, UAB Comprehensive Stroke Center, 1813 6th Avenue South, UAB Hospital Russell Wing, Suite 226, Birmingham, AL 35249.
E-mail address: annealex@uab.edu (A.W. Wojner Alexandrov).

Crit Care Nurs Clin N Am 21 (2009) 435–449
doi:10.1016/j.ccell.2009.09.001
0899-5885/09/$ – see front matter © 2009 Elsevier Inc. All rights reserved.

or, in some cases, highly experienced APNs who were originally mentored by physicians. Although these methods are effective, they fail to standardize learning content, vary in their ability to measure knowledge and skill integration, and are often highly dependent on the expertise and individual initiative of mentors and mentees.

The *Neurovascular Education and Training in Stroke Management and Acute Reperfusion Therapy* (NET SMART) APN program offers a first-of-its-kind, academic, postgraduate, fellowship program for APNs that is modeled after physician academic fellowship programs but supported by a flexible Internet-based platform. This article details the rationale, methods, and preliminary results of the NET SMART APN experience, which serves as a unique template for the development of academic postgraduate nursing fellowship programs across a variety of specialty practices.

PRACTICE SPECIALIZATION METHODS
Advanced Practice Nursing Programs

Nurse practitioners
The first NP program was developed at the University of Colorado in 1965 by a nurse, Dr Loretta Ford, and a physician, Dr Henry Silver. The program sought to alleviate shortages of primary care providers in rural and urban areas. The first NP role was that of a pediatric NP, which focused on health promotion and community health issues.[1] Early NP programs were certificate based, with various entry-level requirements; during the 1970s, an increasing number of NP specialties were recognized, and the first NP certification examination was offered by the American Nurses Association in 1977.[2–7]

In the 1980s, education for NPs shifted from certificate programs to graduate nursing education culminating in a master's degree in nursing with NP specialization. By the end of the 1980s, almost 90% of NP programs were master's degree or post–master's degree certificate programs. During the 1990s, the number of NPs grew exponentially, and the NP role also expanded.[2,4,7] The acute care NP specialty was developed in 1990 to respond to the needs of patients and their families during acute illnesses,[7,8] and NPs became more prevalent in the hospital setting in response to health care's increasing fiscal crisis during the late 1990s.[2,7]

Clinical nurse specialists
The first master's degree program for CNSs was developed in 1954 in response to the rapid emergence of clinical specialty knowledge, incorporation of sophisticated technology into clinical practice, and patient and family needs.[7] This initial program was focused on psychiatry, but the CNS role quvickly spread to maternal-child health, oncology, and cardiac and critical care nursing. In the 1970s, master's degree programs emerged for CNSs in critical care.[7,9–12]

Role confusion has surrounded the CNS position for several years. Contributors to this problem include inappropriate titling as a CNS by nurses who are not graduate-prepared specialists and significant role variability. Realignment of the role to ensure increased practice visibility, coupled with solid practice specialty expertise and a focus on health outcomes management in the 1990s, significantly strengthened role performance and perceived value while placing CNSs in a powerful position to improve interdisciplinary practice.[13] Today, there is recognition of the importance of the CNS role to support evidence-based practice assessment and management.

Advanced practice nurses and neuroscience nursing
There is an emerging presence of CNSs and NPs in neuroscience nursing. A 2006 survey of the APN membership of the American Association of Neuroscience Nurses

revealed that 58.5% of the 282 respondents identified themselves as NPs, whereas 41.5% identified themselves as CNSs.[14] Because there are no graduate APN programs that focus exclusively on entry-level neuroscience education or knowledge, APNs entering this specialty field must bring with them prerequisite knowledge or undergo significant on-the-job training.

Advanced Practice Certification

Professional society generalist and specialty certification serves as a mechanism to ensure safe nursing practice at graduate and undergraduate levels.[15,16] For APNs, graduate academic education is required for licensure or titling in the United States, with many states also requiring professional society certification to support APN titling. The American Nurses Credentialing Center (ANCC) provides APN generalist certification for NPs in adult acute care, adult primary care, family primary care, gerontology primary care, pediatric primary care, and school nursing; ANCC NP specialty certifications include adult psychiatric mental health, diabetes management, and family psychiatric mental health. The ANCC also provides CNS generalist certification in adult health, gerontology, and pediatrics, with specialty certifications that include adult psychiatric mental health, child/adolescent psychiatric mental health, diabetes management, home health, and public/community health. Several other professional nursing organizations also offer APN certification, such as the American Academy of Nurse Practitioners (NP generalist certification), the American Association of Critical-Care Nurses (NP and CNS specialty certification), and the Oncology Nursing Society (CNS specialty certification). No specialty certification exists to support APNs working in the neurosciences or, in particular, advanced neurovascular nursing practice.

Impact of the Advanced Practice Registered Nurse Regulatory Model on Practice Specialization

Uniformity across all US states has been lacking in the definition of APN educational requirements within graduate nursing programs, and licensing and credentialing requirements.[16] Recently, leading professional nursing organizations came together to form the Advanced Practice Registered Nurse (APRN) Consensus Work Group; the group collaborated with the National Council of State Boards of Nursing to develop a framework for requirements supporting APN licensure, graduate APN program accreditation, professional certification, and education for all APRNs.[15] The APRN specialty model (**Fig. 1**) requires that APNs be certified and licensed at the level of one of the four APRN roles (nurse anesthetist, nurse midwife, CNS, or NP) and within at least one of the six populations (family, adult, neonatal, pediatric, women's health, or psychiatry/mental health). Specialization is seen as occurring beyond the scope of the APRN framework, with specialty certification provided by specialist professional nursing organizations.[16]

The APRN regulatory model provides a framework for standardizing APN education within graduate academic nursing programs but precludes provision of education and training in specialty practice in favor of a broad generalist approach. Advantages to the APRN model of generalist education/training include academic content consistency, cross-state portability of APN licensure, a limit on the content depth and time requirements for curriculum completion, and simpler faculty competencies or expertise. APNs who plan to enter specialty practices beyond the scope of the APRN framework, however, require a significant amount of additional education/training to achieve practice competency. Development of postgraduate fellowships across a wide variety of APN specialty practice areas would serve to standardize

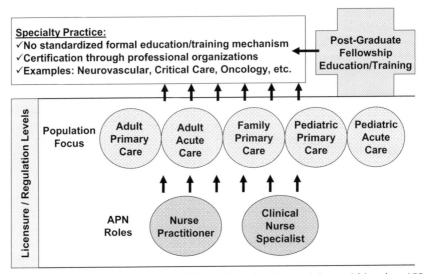

Fig. 1. Positioning of postgraduate fellowship education/training within the APRN regulatory model framework.

preparation of APNs to safely and expertly assume roles in diverse highly specialized practices (see **Fig. 1**).

Physician Specialty Education/Training as a Model for Postgraduate Advanced Practice Nursing Specialty Fellowships

The Accreditation Council for Graduate Medical Education (ACGME) is a nonprofit private council responsible for the accreditation of postgraduate medical training programs (internships, residencies, and fellowships).[17] Accreditation requirements for medical education/training are evaluated against standards addressing the following seven areas:

1. Institution: quality of the sponsoring institution and participating sites
2. Program personnel and resources: quality of the program director, faculty, and other program personnel and resources and medical information access
3. Resident appointments
4. Education program: curricular components, patient care, medical knowledge, practice-based learning and improvement, interpersonal and communication skills, professionalism, systems-based practice, and residents' scholarly activity
5. Evaluation: methods supporting resident formative evaluation, resident summative evaluation, faculty evaluation, and program evaluation and improvement
6. Duty hours: methods for supervision and fatigue prevention and detection, duty hours, on-call activities, and policies for moonlighting and duty hours exceptions
7. Experimentation and innovation[17]

ACGME physician fellowships typically consist of 1 to 2 years of additional specialty education/training completed after successful attainment of generalist board certification within a specific practice focus (eg, general neurology).[17] Fellowship education/training is not uniformly required to provide care to specific specialty patient populations but may be a requirement stipulated in the bylaws of some practice sites. Physicians who chose this degree of specialization are most commonly employed at university-affiliated medical centers that house fellowship education/training programs.

Neurology education/training includes a 4-year residency, of which the first year consists of internal medicine, followed by 3 years of neurology. Neurology postgraduate fellowships may then be entered by interested/eligible candidates in one or more specialty practice areas, including vascular neurology (stroke), interventional neuroradiology, epilepsy, neuromuscular disorders, neurorehabilitation, behavioral neurology, sleep medicine, pain management, neuroimmunology, clinical neurophysiology, or movement disorders. There is typically a 6-month contiguous education/training and validation requirement that supports completion of most physician fellowships, preventing concurrent work outside the selected fellowship program once enrolled.[17]

The seven ACGME fellowship program components provide a model that may be adapted to support APN specialty education/training as follows:

1. Institution: The sponsoring institution and all participating sites must demonstrate that they have access to a large number of patients affected by the diagnosis addressed by the specialty.
2. Program personnel and resources: The program director, faculty, and other program personnel must demonstrate current engagement in the specialty practice at the expert level, in a role that consists of practitioner and researcher elements; resources should include practice facilities that provide high-volume, cutting edge medical/nursing management, with access to advanced patient care technologies, library, and support provided through case- or simulation-based learning methods.
3. Fellowship appointments: APNs must be granted "fellow" status within the program institution, with clearly defined roles and privileges.
4. Education program: Curricular components should be structured in a logical manner that builds on previous learning and encompasses a specialty area of advanced practice knowledge; clinical skills activities that support curricular content must be specified at the direct patient application level to reinforce learning; content should blend medical knowledge, practice-based learning, and improvement with advanced nursing knowledge; mechanisms must be incorporated to promote interpersonal communication skills and professionalism; an understanding of systems-based components in relation to the specialty practice area must be included; and participation in scholarly activities that support knowledge generation, dissemination, and use must be present.
5. Evaluation: Mechanisms for fellow formative and summative evaluation must be established; faculty and program evaluation must be planned for and formally implemented at specified points in time; evaluation data must be aggregated and used for ongoing program improvement; and graduate fellow and faculty outcomes must reflect program mission and values.
6. Duty hours: Specific methods to account for fellow didactic and clinical learning hours must be developed; mechanisms governing local and on-site supervision by qualified practitioner faculty are established; reporting systems for measurement of safe practice are established within local practice sites; and mechanisms governing conduct of fellows during on-site clinical validation must be implemented.
7. Experimentation and innovation: Opportunities for participation in experimental and innovative practice methods must be incorporated into the fellowship experience to foster value and knowledge of evolving scientific and administrative and clinical methods.

THE ARGUMENT FOR ACUTE NEUROVASCULAR ADVANCED PRACTICE NURSING SPECIALIZATION

Stroke is the third most common cause of death in most countries and the leading cause of adult disability; within the neurosciences, stroke consistently ranks as the top admitting diagnosis in most hospitals worldwide.[18] As a vascular disease, stroke possesses a similar risk factor profile to other cardiovascular diseases and, in the case of ischemic stroke, often similar pathogenic mechanisms. Despite data that support the prevalence of stroke, resources capable of ensuring uniform expertise for APNs in the prevention, diagnosis, and treatment of neurovascular disease are seriously lacking.

The initiation of primary stroke center (PSC) certification by The Joint Commission (TJC) has served as a catalyst for US hospitals to adopt evidence-based acute stroke services and, in several US states, TJC certification is required by law for hospitals that admit acute stroke patients. The PSC movement has significantly increased the numbers of interdisciplinary staff with neurovascular learning needs, but few resources currently exist to support the evolution of stroke practice specialization.

Despite achievement of TJC PSC status in more than 600 US hospitals,[19] national tissue-type plasminogen activator (tPA) treatment rates remain extremely low due to a number of factors, including

1. Failure to engage local communities in the early recognition of stroke warning signs and, when available, use of emergency transport systems for rapid transport to a PSC
2. Inconsistent prehospital care operational standards that may foster long on-scene time or failure to recognize stroke warning signs
3. Transfer of suspected acute stroke patients by emergency medical systems personnel to hospitals that do not offer acute stroke treatment (tPA or intra-arterial rescue)
4. Disorganization within emergency departments (EDs) that precludes early diagnosis and treatment of acute stroke patients
5. Limited numbers of fellowship-trained vascular neurologists combined with apathy toward acute stroke treatment among general neurologists for whom regular trips to an ED may be viewed as disruptive to outpatient office schedules
6. An approach to stroke diagnostic work-up that is tied to finding reasons "not to treat" acute stroke patients instead of an aggressive paradigm that finds reasons "to treat" acute neurovascular patients
7. Failure to recognize, educate/train, and implement APNs as diagnosticians, process facilitators, and treatment decision makers in acute neurovascular emergency care

THE NET SMART ADVANCED PRACTICE NURSING POSTGRADUATE FELLOWSHIP PROGRAM
Origins of the Program

In the late 1990s to early 2000s, James Grotta, MD, Professor, Chairman of Neurology, and Director of the University of Texas-Houston Stroke Team, became the first US physician to recognize the value of postgraduate neurovascular fellowship education/training for APNs, providing individualized training while significantly expanding the roles and responsibilities of three nurses (Anne Alexandrov, Robin Saiki, and Dawn Meyer). Grotta's efforts resulted in a high rate of diagnostic agreement between neurologists and APN fellows, safe tPA treatment delivery, and provision of sound hemodynamic management and secondary prevention.

From this experience, Alexandrov later conducted needs assessments targeting APNs, physicians, and hospital administrators to determine their interest in a standardized, evidence-based, neurovascular, postgraduate APN fellowship and their willingness to expand the role of appropriately educated/trained APNs to include the acute diagnosis and management of stroke. Findings indicated significant interest in this expanded role, coupled with the need for flexible access to learning materials to ensure availability and feasibility of the program. These data, coupled with Health Resources and Services Administration funding, supported the genesis of the NET SMART APN fellowship program, which to date has enrolled more than 70 neurovascular APN fellows.

Overview of the Program

The principle target outcome of the NET SMART program is to develop a critical mass of APNs capable of providing neurovascular clinical practice leadership that results in improved tPA treatment rates and patient and hospital outcomes. To achieve this outcome, a systematic approach to neurovascular education and training was developed using an on-line platform that is accessible 24 hours per day, 7 days per week, and 365 days per year and easily updated based on emerging scientific findings. **Table 1** presents the NET SMART APN curriculum, which consists of 14 modules that progress from primary prevention to emergency systems, acute assessment and diagnosis, reperfusion therapies, evolving treatment methods, neurocritical care, complication avoidance measures, secondary prevention, stroke center leadership, APN role innovation, and entry into rehabilitation. Because NET SMART's mission is closely tied to acute stroke diagnosis and treatment, significant emphasis is placed on acute care management, whereas rehabilitation concepts are introduced but not elaborated on to a significant degree.

Criteria for enrollment into the NET SMART APN fellowship include master's degree preparation as a NP or clinical specialist or current graduate student status within 12 months of program completion. Mechanisms exist to support students enrolled in master's of nursing or doctor of nursing practice programs, including the ability to use NET SMART program time as elective or practice hours with the approval of local faculty. Recently, enrollment was expanded to include master's degree–prepared nurses without an APN role focus (eg, nursing education or administration), although a requirement for at least part-time practice in a related neurovascular role (eg, stroke coordinator or nurse manager) is required.

Enrolled fellows must contract with a local physician supervisor, preferably a neurologist, to provide oversight for clinical skills training and support ongoing learning. In the absence of local neurologist support, fellows may contract with a combination of physician providers, including neurosurgeons, emergency physicians, cardiologists, and radiologists; program faculty also work closely with fellows who do not have local neurologist support to ensure an appropriate learning environment is provided. Fellows also must provide evidence of administrative support for their role, including a willingness to provide data that support process and outcomes measurement during and after program completion, to allow assessment of program metrics.

NET SMART modules are supported by comprehensive testing delivered in a pretest/post-test manner to foster assessment of learning needs and a shift in knowledge. Modular content is deliberately leveled to that of a vascular neurology physician fellowship, with the expectation that APN fellows can articulate findings from all key clinical trials and integrate these findings into practice locally in their

Table 1
NET SMART curriculum (course content in sequence)

Course Title	Description
Module 1: Introduction to acute stroke	This introductory module reviews stroke typology and pathophysiology, methods for clinical trial design in stroke and evidence quality, findings from pivotal epidemiologic studies in stroke, common risk factors for stroke, and assignment of pathogenic mechanism: I. Introduction of stroke typology II. Introduction to clinical trial design in stroke III. Significant studies in stroke epidemiology IV. Risk factor assessment and incidence V. Determination of stroke pathogenic mechanism
Module 2: Emergency systems for acute stroke patients—prehospital, triage, and emergency department management	This module reviews guideline-based recommendations for stroke systems of care, along with examples from highly successful programs. Mechanisms to engage widespread community involvement in acute stroke prevention, early recognition and emergent transport for treatment are presented: I. Prehospital systems for acute stroke—protocols, algorithms, preferential transport, and communication mechanisms II. Field and departmental triage of stroke emergencies III. Emergency assessment: priorities, quality measures, and practitioner/systems alignment IV. Laboratory diagnostics for treatment decision making V. Innovative telemedicine and prehospital emergency assessment/management approaches VI. Engaging the community in stroke prevention and recognition VII. Legislative efforts for stroke
Module 3: Clinical localization of stroke: Integrated anatomy, physiology, and assessment	This module provides fellows with an understanding of the anatomy and physiology of the central nervous system in relation to signs and symptoms suggestive of acute stroke. Fellows learn how to clinically localize strokes by the presentation of findings suggestive of particular vascular territories in the brain. The module concludes with a review of standardized stroke scales and how these support ongoing neurologic and functional assessment in stroke: I. Vascular territories of the brain II. Anatomy, physiology, and correlated clinical assessment III. Localizing lesions by clinical examination IV. Standardized stroke scales
Module 4: CT imaging in acute stroke	This module reviews the utility of CT in acute stroke. Anatomic correlation on CT and ischemic and hemorrhagic stroke imaging findings are presented: I. Introduction to CT II. Guide to interpretation of CT III. Differentiation of lesions by clinical correlates and imaging vascular distribution IV. Distinguishing hemorrhage from ischemia V. Hypodensities and changes associated with ischemia VI. Imaging priorities in transient ischemic attack

(continued on next page)

Table 1
(continued)

Course Title	Description
Module 5: MRI imaging in acute stroke	This module reviews the utility of MRI in acute stroke. Fellows learn different MRI sequences (localizer, TI, T2, diffusion-weighted imaging, fluid-attenuated inversion recovery, perfusion-weighted imaging, gradient-recalled echo imaging, and apparent diffusion coefficient) and are introduced to anatomic correlates: I. Introduction to MRI II. Guide to interpretation of MRI III. Differentiation of lesions by clinical correlates and imaging vascular distribution IV. Distinguishing hemorrhage from ischemic changes V. Transient ischemic attack imaging
Module 6: Multimodal angiographic imaging	This module explores multimodal angiography techniques, including the use of CT angiography and CT perfusion, magnetic resonance angiography, and digital subtraction angiography: I. Introduction to multimodal angiographic techniques II. Guide to interpretation of angiography III. Limitations of angiographic approaches
Module 7: Ultrasound (carotid and vertebral duplex, TCD) in acute stroke	This module covers use of ultrasound testing in acute stroke in relation to other imaging modalities and determination of pathogenic mechanism and secondary prevention needs: I. Utility of ultrasound in acute stroke management II. Transcranial Doppler applications in emergent assessment, reperfusion monitoring, and long-term patient management III. Carotid duplex and vertebrobasilar assessment of stroke etiology IV. Ultrasound as a complimentary modality to MRI, CT, and angiography
Module 8: Indications for and administration of reperfusion therapy	This module covers current evidence-based guidelines supporting reperfusion therapy with intravenous tPA and evolving indications and techniques for intra-arterial rescue therapies. Fellows learn indications, dosages, and common pitfalls in administration of thrombolytic treatment for stroke: I. Reperfusion methods and treatment selection II. Reperfusion sequela: prevention and detection of intracranial hemorrhage III. Oropharyngeal edema: airway protection and treatment options IV. Monitoring recanalization and clinical improvement V. Concurrent management of blood pressure
Module 9: Management of intracranial hemorrhage and neurocritical care for stroke	This module covers current and experimental approaches to the management of intracranial hemorrhage while introducing fellows to concepts central to the management of neurocritical care stroke patients: I. Introduction to management of intraparenchymal and subarachnoid hemorrhage II. Common neurocritical care procedures and practices for ischemic and hemorrhagic stroke III. Emerging aggressive management regimes: craniectomy, hypothermia, and hemodynamic augmentation

(continued on next page)

Table 1
(continued)

Course Title	Description
Module 10: Complications of stroke—prevention, recognition, and management	Major and common complications of ischemic and hemorrhagic strokes are reviewed along with the protocols for monitoring, detection, and treatment to prevent those complications. Special emphasis is paid to aspiration pneumonia, skin breakdown, contractures, deep vein thrombosis, poststroke depression, urinary tract infections, and the newly described reversed Robin Hood syndrome: I. Risk factors for stroke-related complications II. Prevention, from field through hospital management III. Early recognition of complications IV. Medical and nursing management of complications
Module 11: Secondary stroke prevention	Early institution of secondary stroke prevention treatment and discharge on appropriate medications is reviewed. Compliance issues and current indications for the use of specific agents are discussed: I. Physiologic actions and selection of antithrombotic agents II. Statins for secondary prevention III. Glucose control IV. Smoking cessation
Module 12: Stroke units—TJC PSC certification and comprehensive stroke center framework	Content is presented on stroke unit organization, including methods to reconfigure existing space, staffing, and work process. Preparation for TJC certification as a PSC is discussed, and fellows are introduced to a framework for comprehensive stroke center designation: I. Inside the stroke unit: system requirements for optimal organization II. Common stroke unit models for staffing and practice: protocols, pathways and algorithmic care III. Outcomes of stroke unit management: defining successful process and outcome interaction IV. Aligning Brain Attack Coalition and American Stroke Association guidelines with TJC certification processes. V. Assessing readiness for certification and constructing the certification application VI. Promoting staff readiness: educational tools and conducting a mock survey VII. Brain Attack Coalition guidelines as a framework for comprehensive stroke center designation
Module 13: Innovative methods for stroke center operations: use of APNs; stroke center quality improvement: stroke registries and repositories	This course presents content on innovative approaches to quality management of stroke programs, including use of APNs to support a stroke center endeavor, integration of electronic medical record processes into the quality program, and methods to build support through staff ownership of overall program quality: I. Practice models for stroke center APNs: program regulations, credentialing, and APN responsibilities II. Personal practice improvement strategies: measuring quality and initiating research III. Teleradiology and telemedicine systems for APN practice in acute stroke IV. Quality requirements for stroke centers V. Registries, electronic health records, and institution-specific data repositories VI. Engaging interdisciplinary staff in quality and research efforts

(continued on next page)

Course Title	Description
Table 1 (*continued*)	

Module 14:
  Neurorehabilitation
  and recovery
	This module covers evaluation of candidates for rehabilitation, early initiation of physical/speech/occupational therapy, and cutting-edge rehabilitation strategies:
	I. Rehabilitation begins in acute care
	II. Regulatory and system requirements for rehabilitative placement
	III. Nursing assessment of readiness and need
	IV. Collaborative initiation of rehabilitation

On-site clinical preceptorship	The 80-hour clinical preceptorship focuses on validation of content learned during completion of the NET SMART modules. Participants complete several clinical rotations and experiences with expert clinical practitioners and receive ongoing performance feedback

practice sites. To accomplish this, the introductory module incorporates in-depth content on clinical trials design and levels of evidence, whereas later modules build on understanding and application of this introductory material. Module lectures are delivered using Adobe Breeze technology that provides audio lectures along with Microsoft PowerPoint slides and video to enhance learning.

Fig. 2 presents an overview of program progression. Each of the 14 modules is accompanied by clinical skills activities that ensure clinical application of knowledge to practice. Fellows complete activities under the supervision of their local physician supervisors and submit their work for grading to a program coordinator. After completion of modular lecture content and clinical skills activities, the post-test for the module must be passed before advancing to the next module. All modules are externally reviewed by leaders in vascular neurology for content accuracy, relevance, and comprehensiveness.

After successful completion of all 14 modules, fellows advance to an on-site clinical validation session, which is provided at the University of Alabama at Birmingham, Comprehensive Stroke Center. The session consists of 80 hours of supervised clinical time within this fast-paced, high stroke–volume hospital located in the "stroke belt" region of the United States. While on site, fellows are provided with beepers to alert them to acute stroke admissions and are expected to round daily in the hospital with the stroke team, including responding to all code stroke events and seeing patients post discharge in the stroke clinic. Specific competencies validated during the experience include

- Ability to accurately interpret neuroimaging (CT, MRI, angiography, and Doppler-based images)
- Ability to clinically localize physical examination findings to discrete neurovascular territories
- Ability to safely recommend prescription of acute stroke treatment (tPA and intra-arterial rescue)
- Ability to provide safe, evidence-based medical and nursing management recommendations for ischemic and hemorrhagic stroke
- Ability to work effectively across several acute stroke settings, including ED, neurocritical care unit, stroke unit, and stroke clinic
- Ability to appropriately work-up and accurately assign stroke pathogenic mechanism

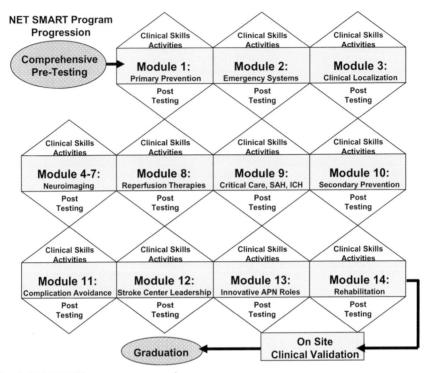

Fig. 2. NET SMART program progression.

- Ability to appropriately recommend prescription of prophylaxis or treatment for secondary prevention of stroke in accordance with pathogenic mechanism and risk factor profile
- Ability to assess needs and recommend prescription of methods for complication avoidance
- Ability to provide stroke program leadership as a specialist APN
- Ability to articulate the relationship between clinical research findings and recommended medical and nursing therapies
- Ability to integrate advanced nursing practice into medical management of acute neurovascular patients.

Preliminary Program Outcomes

Pretesting of NET SMART fellows indicates significant learning needs among even the most experienced APNs in all program areas, with post-test scores and clinical skills assignments demonstrating significant knowledge growth and competency development. Program outcomes to date demonstrate a 7% increase in the rate of intravenous tPA treatment among fellows' local practice sites compared with baseline reported rates, and several sites have gone on to attain TJC PSC certification under NET SMART fellow leadership. Local physician supervisors indicate a significant increase in fellow knowledge and practice competency and a high degree of satisfaction with fellow performance. Several local physicians admit to learning alongside their fellows by viewing module content on-line.

Program completion time is largely self-paced, although fellows with slow progression are regularly encouraged to pick up the pace of their learning. Responsibilities that fellows cite as being added to their roles since the time of NET SMART enrollment include first-responder duties for all code strokes, preliminary interpretation of neuro-imaging findings, prescribing intravenous tPA for treatment of ischemic stroke, intraprocedural management of intra-arterial rescue cases, stroke program leadership, and supervision of medical residents on neurovascular rotations. While credentialing and privileging are dependent on local practice site regulations, scope of practice, and local medical politics, the addition of these responsibilities is promising and serves to position these fellowship-educated APNs in positions that may dramatically improve acute stroke outcomes. For nonprescribing APNs and stroke coordinators, the additional knowledge gained in the fellowship has enabled these nurses to work more effectively through their local neurologists and other physicians providing stroke care. Despite an inability to prescribe tPA or other therapies, these fellows are able to oversee care, expertly localize lesions to neurovascular territory, interpret neuroimaging, communicate findings, cite evidence-based rationale for recommended therapies, and stimulate physician action to treat and prevent acute stroke. Combined, prescribing and nonprescribing fellows are well suited to improve acute stroke care and the impact of stroke burden in their communities.

NET SMART Through the Eyes of Advanced Practice Nursing Fellows

NET SMART fellows are mavericks who have embarked on a first-of-its-kind learning journey and describe the experience as empowering for APNs. Fellows cite outcomes that include improved practice confidence, improved physician-APN relationships, improved physician trust in APN diagnostic judgment and management, recognition of APN neurovascular expertise among different physician specialties (eg, emergency medicine and internal medicine), respect for the neurovascular APN role, and expanded autonomy in role performance. Also valued is the camaraderie and networking that develops among fellows, especially during the on-site clinical validation experience, which brings fellows together from across the country. Fellows learn that they often share challenges and frustrations in their local practice sites that may be solved through shared dialog that promotes collaborative problem solving. Specific strengths of the NET SMART program cited by fellows include

- Authentic practice and research expertise among program faculty
- Accessibility of program faculty throughout the distance learning process
- Distance learning accessibility
- Ability to become immersed in an aggressive treatment philosophy that can challenge local treatment paradigms
- Provision of regular performance feedback
- Clinical exercises that ensure application of new knowledge
- Culmination of the experience in a high-volume, complex, aggressive stroke center, which enables a look at how things are done at other centers
- Esprit de corps among fellows and faculty
- Networking among fellows and faculty
- Regularly updated, evidence-based content
- Expectations for fellows to be able to clearly articulate how clinical trials drive changes in practice

RECOMMENDATIONS FOR ADVANCED PRACTICE NURSING FELLOWSHIPS

Organization of APN fellowship programs is not suited to all organizations. APN fellows are a highly motivated and experienced group of clinicians capable of easily spotting imposter faculty who lack practical expertise or are solely dependent on theoretic knowledge. APN fellows also expect a significant degree of expert practice immersion, which necessitates clinical experiences that add value (not busy work), are relevant, and are tied to important practice competencies. Faculty intent on developing an APN fellowship must honestly reflect their ability to mentor this elite group of clinicians.

The hub practice site sponsoring an APN fellowship must also be closely considered, as it reflects the credibility of the program. The site must be recognized for provision of cutting-edge, evidence-based medical and nursing practice; supported by world class, well-recognized, attending physicians and attending nurse leaders; and seen as a leader in the evolution of clinical science for the specialty practice. Collectively, the credibility of a practice site and its faculty will drive the success of any APN fellowship program.

A significant amount of time must be set aside to develop and revise learning materials. Program content must be regularly evaluated against evolving scientific findings. This necessitates attendance at all key scientific meetings worldwide, regular journal scanning for new findings in need of inclusion, and networking with key interdisciplinary practice leaders throughout the world. In the authors' experience, more than 70% of program modules require updating at least every 6 months to maintain their relevancy and accuracy.

Other considerations include an Internet platform to provide the program, because on-line offerings enhance access worldwide. Manpower considerations include the need for personnel to maintain the on-line systems, including Web site updates. Graphic design personnel are also needed to assist with program branding, logo design, and development of original art that supports learning. A program coordinator is necessary to work directly with fellows and assist with registration, program statistics, and program matriculation. A researcher specializing in psychometric analyses should also be contracted, to ensure ongoing evaluation and improvement of test items. Key thought leaders in the specialty should be consulted to assist with regular program content assessment and provide recommendations for revision. Lastly, mechanisms must also be developed to support program marketing, including exhibiting at conferences, direct mailing, Web site positioning, and journal advertisement.

SUMMARY

Acute neurovascular patients remain significantly underserved due to a combination of stroke physician shortages and physician disinterest in acute stroke treatment. Postgraduate neurovascular fellowship–trained APNs are well positioned to improve stroke patient and hospital outcomes while furthering the role of specialty educated/trained nurses.

NET SMART APN serves as a model for postgraduate APN fellowship education and training. Faculty and institutions capable of providing specialty-level APN programs across a wide variety of specialty areas are encouraged take on this charge to promote standardization of evidence-based content and learning methods that will further the role APNs may play within healthcare settings for years to come.

ACKNOWLEDGMENTS

The authors wish to acknowledge the support of Tenisha Baca, Program Coordinator, and Stephen DiBiase, Graphic Designer and Web Master for their significant contributions to the NETSMART program.

REFERENCES

1. Carnegie Commission on Higher Education. Quality and equality: new levels of federal responsibility for higher education. New York: Carnegie Commission; 1968.
2. Asubonteng P, McCleary KF, Munchus G. Nurse practitioners in the USA—their past, present and future: some implications for the health care management delivery system. Health Manpow Manage 1995;21(3):3–10.
3. DiCenso A. Roles, research and resilience: the evolution of advanced practice nursing. Can Nurse 2008;104(9):37–40.
4. Bear EM. Advanced practice nurses: how did we get here anyway? Adv Pract Nurs Q 1995;1(1):10–4.
5. Alexander M, Walters H, Noordenbos A. Controversial, confident and committed: how a close knit group of believers launched the NP profession. Interview with Jolynn Tumolo. Adv Nurse Pract 2005;13(5):53–4.
6. Por J. A critical engagement with the concept of advancing nursing practice. J Nurs Manag 2008;16(1):84–90.
7. Coombs M, Chaboyer W, Sole ML. Advanced nursing roles in critical care—a natural or forced evolution? J Prof Nurs 2007;23(2):83–90.
8. American Nurses Association. Standards of clinical practice and scope of practice for the Acute Care Nurse Practitioner. Washington, DC: American Nurses Association and American Association of Critical Care Nurses; 1995.
9. Lindeke LL, Canedy BH, Kay MM. A comparison of practice domains of clinical nurse specialists and nurse practitioners. J Prof Nurs 1997;13(5):281–7.
10. Dunn L. A literature review of advanced clinical nursing practice in the United States of America. J Adv Nurs 1997;25(4):814–9.
11. LaSalla CA, Connors PM, Pedro JT, et al. The role of the clinical nurse specialist in promoting evidence-based practice and effecting positive patient outcomes. J Contin Educ Nurs 2007;38(6):262–70.
12. Hanson CM, Hamric AB. Reflections on the continuing evolution of advanced practice nursing. Nurs Outlook 2003;51(5):203–11.
13. Wojner AW. Outcomes management: application to clinical practice. St Louis (MO): Mosby; 2001.
14. Villanueva N, Blank-Reid C, Stewart-Amidei C, et al. The role of the advanced practice nurse in neuroscience nursing: results of the 2006 AANN membership survey. J Neurosci Nurs 2008;40(2):119–24.
15. Stanley J. Reaching consensus on a regulatory model: what does this mean for APRNs? J Nurse Pract 2009;5(2):99–104.
16. APRN Consensus Work Group & National Council of State Boards of Nursing APRN Advisory Committee. Consensus Model for APRN Regulation: licensure, accreditation, certification & education. Available at: http://www.aacn.nche.edu. Accessed December 10, 2008.
17. Accreditation Council for Graduate Medical Education. Accreditation standards for specialty fellowship education/training. Available at: http://www.acgme.org/acWebsite/home/home.asp. Accessed July 22, 2009.
18. Alberts MJ, Hademenos G, Latchaw RE, et al. Recommendations for the establishment of primary stroke centers. JAMA 2000;283:3102–9.
19. The Joint Commission. Disease-specific care: primary stroke center certification. Available at: http://www.jointcommission.org. Accessed July 22, 2009.

Hyperacute Ischemic Stroke Management: Reperfusion and Evolving Therapies

Anne W. Wojner Alexandrov, PhD, RN, CCRN, FAAN[a,b,c,*]

KEYWORDS

- Ischemic stroke • Tissue plasminogen activator (tPA)
- Intra-arterial rescue procedures • Reperfusion therapies

Management of acute ischemic stroke patients is organized around several priorities aimed at ensuring optimal patient outcomes. The first priority is provision of reperfusion therapies aimed at recanalization of obstructed arterial vessels, thereby restoring brain perfusion and minimizing disability. Following reperfusion therapy, or in patients that lack an indication for reperfusion therapy, priorities shift to determination of pathogenic mechanism by provision of a comprehensive workup to determine probable cause of the ischemic stroke (or transient ischemic attack [TIA]), for the purpose of providing appropriate prophylaxis (secondary prevention) for subsequent events. Provision of secondary prevention measures along with therapies that prevent complications associated with neurologic disability, and evaluation for the most appropriate level of rehabilitation services become the final priorities during acute hospitalization.

This article provides an overview of reperfusion therapies and emerging hemodynamic treatments for hyperacute ischemic strokes. Gaps in the scientific evidence that are driving current blood flow augmentation research are identified.

HYPERACUTE STROKE MANAGEMENT
Prehospital Evaluation and Management

Although systems and personnel requirements vary, most regions in North America offer some system of emergency response, stabilization, and transport of patients to hospitals for definitive diagnosis and treatment. In acute stroke, use of valid and reliable prehospital stroke scales such as the Cincinnati Prehospital Stroke Scale or the Los Angeles Prehospital Stroke Scale have been shown to improve accuracy in the

[a] Acute & Critical Care, School of Nursing, USA
[b] Vascular Neurology, School of Medicine, USA
[c] Comprehensive Stroke Center, University of Alabama, Birmingham 35249, USA
* Comprehensive Stroke Center, University of Alabama, Birmingham 35249, USA.
E-mail address: annealex@uab.edu

Crit Care Nurs Clin N Am 21 (2009) 451–470
doi:10.1016/j.ccell.2009.08.001
0899-5885/09/$ – see front matter © 2009 Elsevier Inc. All rights reserved.

recognition of stroke patients.[1-3] Application of prehospital standardized protocols further benefits prehospital care by outlining care priorities, limiting the time spent on scene, and expediting the rapid direct transport of suspected stroke patients to hospitals capable of delivering acute stroke treatment.[3-9] These measures collectively are tied to increasing the number of stroke patients eligible for receiving reperfusion therapies.

Emergency Evaluation and Management

Within the Emergency Department (ED), interdisciplinary staff must also remain alert to recognition of acute stroke patients, because regional limitations in ambulance transportation or knowledge deficits among lay persons contribute to a significant number of acute stroke patients arriving by private car.[9-14] Use of simple scales such as the Cincinnati Prehospital Stroke Scale[2] in the triage area of the ED may result in rapid identification of patients with findings suggestive of an acute stroke or TIA.

Emergency triage of an acute stroke or TIA patient using the Emergency Severity Index typically falls into category 2 (**Fig. 1**), although category 1 may also be selected in cases presenting with concurrent airway breathing or hemodynamic instability.[15,16] All suspected stroke or TIA patients, with or without current neurologic deficit, should be rapidly identified in the triage area and immediately admitted for diagnosis and, if indicated, reperfusion therapy. Determining the time of stroke symptom onset or the time the patient was last seen as normal is a high priority for triage personnel.

To accomplish efficient emergency management of suspected stroke patients, most EDs have implemented standing orders that empower nurses to institute care before an initial assessment by an emergency physician. Along with assessment and management of airway (A), breathing (B), and circulation (C), coupled with a *brief*

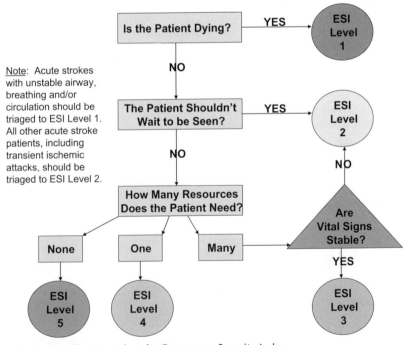

Fig. 1. Stroke classification using the Emergency Severity Index.

primary neurologic disability (D) assessment, these independent nursing measures most commonly include:

1. Calling a "Code Stroke" alert in the hospital, so that the Stroke Team is mobilized to come to the ED
2. Administering 100% oxygen by non-rebreather mask
3. Establishing two 0.9 normal saline intravenous lines
4. Ordering/drawing initial blood work (complete blood count, blood chemistries and glucose, coagulation profile, cardiac enzymes)
5. Ordering a "STAT" noncontrast computed tomography (CT) scan of the head
6. Completing a 12-lead electrocardiogram
7. Ordering an upright portable chest radiograph if indicated by airway or oxygenation assessment findings
8. Completing the National Institutes of Health Stroke Scale (NIHSS)
9. Ordering/collecting a drug screen panel if indicated
10. In the case of patients with significant neurologic disability (eg, decreased level of consciousness, compromised cognitive function, dense hemiplegia), insertion of a urinary catheter

The National Institute for Neurological Disorders and Stroke[17] and the Brain Attack Coalition (BAC) Guidelines[18,19] identify the need for physician evaluation of an acute stroke patient within 10 minutes of arrival to the ED, completion of a noncontrast CT within 25 minutes of hospital arrival, and CT diagnostic interpretation within 45 minutes of hospital arrival (**Fig. 2**). These guidelines are closely adhered to in the most experienced Stroke Centers throughout the world, in keeping with the philosophy that "time is brain." The aim of these guidelines is to facilitate timely administration of reperfusion therapies in appropriate ischemic stroke candidates, so that in the case of treatment with tissue plasminogen activator (tPA), the thrombolytic bolus can be administered within 60 minutes of arrival to the hospital. However, completion of

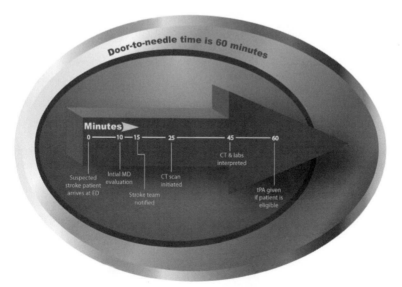

Fig. 2. The "Golden Hour" for tPA treatment. *Courtesy of* Stephen DiBiase Designs, Scottsdale, AZ; with permission.

a thorough workup for tPA treatment candidacy may be sufficiently completed within less than 60 minutes by Stroke Teams that have become expert in their ability to rapidly develop and use systems for accurate diagnosis and treatment delivery. In the case of patients arriving to the hospital with less than 60 minutes left in the intravenous tPA window, the ability for timely, rapid, expert response is paramount to achieving optimal stroke treatment and outcomes. The drive for excellence in the delivery of acute reperfusion therapies has caused many departments to institute an Emergency Stroke Reperfusion Scorecard based on the BAC guidelines (**Fig. 3**) to support ongoing measurement and improvement of their ED systems and processes.

Once ABCs have been assessed, if necessary stabilized, and a quick primary neurologic disability (D) assessment has been performed, rapid progression of the patient to noncontrast CT is paramount.[3] Noncontrast CT is highly sensitive for the presence of blood, allowing practitioners to rapidly identify the presence of hemorrhagic stroke for the purpose of excluding reperfusion therapies from the treatment plan.[3,18,20–22] In the case of hyperacute ischemic stroke (symptoms occurring within 6–8 hours of hospital arrival), the noncontrast CT should be normal or contain only early infarct signs such as sulcal effacement, blurring of the gray/white interface, or a hyperdense artery sign; when this is the case, care progresses to rapid completion of a more focused, structured neurologic examination along with quantification of the neurologic disability by means of a valid and reliable tool, such as the NIHSS.[23–30] Of paramount importance is whether the disability follows neurovascular territory in the brain, which assists with localization of the arterial occlusion.

Use of additional neuroimaging technologies to image vessel occlusion is unnecessary to make a tPA treatment decision, but may complement the diagnostic workup; CT angiography (CTA) and transcranial Doppler (TCD) may be completed rapidly and may increase provider confidence in the diagnosis of ischemic stroke, although it is

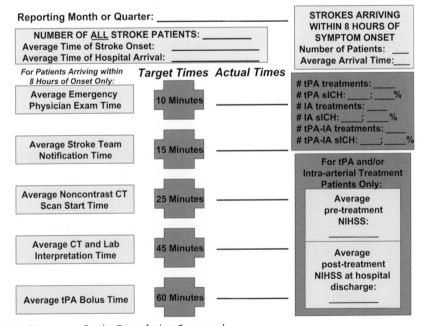

Fig. 3. Emergency Stroke Reperfusion Scorecard.

important to emphasize that small vessel occlusions that warrant treatment with tPA may be missed using these technologies.[3] Use of magnetic resonance imaging (MRI) to assist with the rapid diagnosis and management of stroke is usually impractical, except in advanced Stroke Centers where rapid MRI protocols have been established with short scanning times.[3] In the case of hemorrhagic stroke, intraparenchymal hemorrhages occurring outside a territory suggestive of a hypertensive mechanism should be considered for additional neuroimaging with CTA or catheter angiography, to exclude an aneurysmal or arteriovenous malformation mechanism.[3]

Delivery of Reperfusion Therapies in Hyperacute Ischemic Stroke

Once acute ischemic stroke has been diagnosed, the patient should be positioned with the head of the bed at zero degrees. Flat, zero-degree positioning has been shown to increase blood flow by 20% through the residual arterial lumen affected by stroke[31]; in addition, early (between 0 and 48 hours) development of increased intracranial pressure (ICP) is unlikely in most ischemic stroke patients, making zero-degree positioning an important first step in enhancing perfusion within penumbral territory. Ischemic stroke patients arriving within 180 minutes of symptom onset that meet criteria for tPA treatment should be rapidly thrombolysed with intravenous tPA (IV-tPA),[3,18,19] and at those North American centers (approved in Canada; in the United States, provided as "off-label" use at several comprehensive stroke centers at the time of writing) that have adopted the findings from the European cooperative acute stroke study—3 trial (ECASS-3),[32] the IV-tPA window is extended to 270 minutes from symptom onset. In most United States hospitals, administration of IV-tPA does not require written consent, because patients with acute stroke are viewed to be at significant risk for severe neurologic disability that warrants emergency medical treatment with all available approved therapies; this approach of waived written consent for IV-tPA treatment in ischemic stroke mirrors the expedited management approach that would be applied to major traumatic injury requiring emergency surgery, or a presentation of acute myocardial infarction warranting emergency reperfusion. In addition, because neurologic disability may preclude a stroke patient's ability to sign his or her own written consent, waiting to obtain consent from the legally designated family member may prevent administration of IV-tPA within a timely manner, thereby worsening subsequent neurologic disability.

Numerous studies have demonstrated the safety and benefit of IV-tPA for the treatment of acute ischemic stroke.[32–39] In the hands of well-trained, experienced Stroke Teams, symptomatic intracerebral hemorrhage (sICH), defined as an increase in 4 or more points on the NIHSS associated with a posttreatment finding of hemorrhage on noncontrast CT,[3] is a relatively rare event. In fact, Stroke Teams with high IV-tPA treatment rates typically have sICH rates that are much lower than the 6.4% sICH rate observed in the NIH National Institutes of Neurologic Disorders and Stroke (NINDS) tPA Study[33] that led to national drug approval in the United States in 1996, demonstrating that experience with IV-tPA administration is associated with reduced treatment complications.

It is also important to rationally consider the risk of sICH in relation to the risk of significant neurologic disability. For example, using the data from the NINDS tPA trial,[32] about 6 patients out of 100 treated with IV-tPA may be at risk for development of an sICH; applying the data from the Phase IV European "safe implementation of thrombolysis in stroke monitoring study" (SITS-MOST),[39] about 2 patients (1.7%) out of 100 treated with IV-tPA may be at risk of developing an sICH. In addition, in the NINDS tPA trial,[33] 39% of patients receiving IV-tPA compared with only 26% of placebo patients achieved a modified Rankin Score (mRS) of 0 to 1 by 3 months, and these patients had a 30% greater chance of sustaining either minimal or no neurologic disability at 3 months compared with placebo patients. Of note, SITS-MOST data also demonstrated that 39% of subjects receiving tPA had attained an mRS of 0 to 1 by 3 months,[39] providing significant validation of both the safety and benefit of IV-tPA in the treatment of acute ischemic stroke patients.

The odds of significant neurologic improvement with reduction of devastating neurologic disability clearly outweigh the risks associated with IV-tPA treatment. In fact, where resistance remains to the use of IV-tPA for ischemic stroke, it is likely due to the challenge of updating emergency systems with slow approaches to stroke care, inexperienced practitioners that may be unwilling to take on emergency stroke management, or health systems with significant financial constraints that are incapable of supporting the cost of swift diagnostic imaging, emergency medical/nursing management, and the cost of IV-tPA. However, it is important to recognize that hyperacute stroke practice today equates to "STAT" emergency management, and it is likely to continue down this path for years to come as researchers explore other methods aimed at enhancing or restoring brain perfusion to ward off neurologic disability.

Adherence to an evidence-based protocol for administration of IV-tPA is closely tied to patient outcome. Although optimal, weighing ischemic stroke patients in the ED is rarely undertaken, and was not undertaken in any of the IV-tPA trials. Instead, patients or family are asked to provide approximate weight data, or in the absence of this information, weight is estimated by the Stroke Team. Dosage of IV-tPA is then calculated using the formula:

0.9mgtPA/kg patient weight

The total dose of tPA should never exceed a total of 90 mg, so when the calculated dose exceeds this level it is dropped back to the 90 mg limit. Once the total dose has been calculated, 10% of the total is given as an intravenous bolus over 1 minute; the remaining 90% of the dose is then hung and infused over the next 60 minutes. tPA reconstitution results in 100 mg/100 mL. To ensure accuracy of dose delivered, many recommend withdrawal of the amount *not* to be infused before hanging the vial as follows.

    a. Withdraw with a 10-mL syringe a 10% bolus dose; inject over 1 minute. (Clinical example: if the total dose to be given is 68 mg, the 10% bolus dose amounts to 6.8 mg or 6.8 mL; 93.2 mg remaining in the vial.)

    b. Withdraw the tPA now remaining in the vial that is in excess of the 68 mg total dose. (Clinical example: 68 mg − 6.8 mg = 61.2 mg (61.2 mL); with 93.2 mg remaining in the vial, the Stroke Team nurse should withdraw 32 mL of the reconstituted tPA, leaving only 61.2 mL in the vial for infusion.) The withdrawn tPA can be discarded, or in the case of continuing treatment by intra-arterial rescue, the tPA should be clearly labeled and sent with the interventionalist for use in the catheterization laboratory. Infuse the final 61.2 mg over 60 minutes, ensuring that all tPA remaining in the tubing reaches the patient before the infusion is discontinued.

Before administration of the bolus, as well as throughout the tPA infusion and post-infusion period, it is paramount that blood pressure be precisely and accurately measured and controlled to maintain the parameters noted in **Table 1**.[3] Inability to appropriately control blood pressure is the most common reason associated with sICH in IV-tPA treated patients; all deviations from specified blood pressure

Table 1	
American Stroke Association (2007) guidelines for acute blood pressure management	
If _Treating_ with tPA:	
BP Level (mm Hg)	**Recommended Treatment**

Pretreatment
    SBP >185 or
    DBP >110
	Labetalol 10–20 mg over 1–2 min, or Nitropaste 1–2 in, or
	nicardipine infusion started at 5 mg/h

During & after tPA
    SBP >180
    DBP >105
	Labetalol 10–20 mg over 1–2 min, or nicardipine infusion
	started at 5 mg/h

If _not treating_ with tPA, BP may be left untreated up to SBP 220 mm Hg and DBP 120 mm Hg.
    Abbreviations: BP, blood pressure; DBP, diastolic blood pressure; SBP, systolic blood pressure; tPA, tissue plasminogen activator.

parameters must be immediately acted on with intravenous antihypertensive agents to ensure patient safety. Pharmaceutical agents that allow for rapid, precise, nonaggressive blood pressure reduction are recommended, because significant blood pressure lowering will result in decreased blood flow through the residual arterial lumen, which may worsen perfusion within the ischemic penumbra.[3,40,41]

Use of noninvasive oscillometric automatic blood pressure (NIBP) cuffs had originally been thought to be dangerous in IV-tPA treated patients because of intense mechanical compression of the arm that might facilitate bleeding into soft tissues. However, no study has been undertaken to support this concern, and these devices are regularly used in many facilities without deleterious effects. Whereas one cannot conclude that NIBPs are entirely safe, it also cannot be concluded that they are unsafe; future investigations by nurses may assist in quantifying safety concerns with these devices during and after treatment with IV-tPA.

Elevated glucose levels should also be identified early in the hyperacute phase due to their association with poor neurologic outcome; when present, elevated glucose should be treated with regular insulin before treatment with tPA to achieve a value ranging from 80 to 110 mg/dL.[3,42–45] In addition, the presence of fever in acute stroke patients is also associated with poor outcome, and these patients should be rapidly returned to normothermic levels using routine measures such as acetaminophen or cooling blankets.[3,46–53]

Other nursing priorities during and after delivery of IV-tPA include close monitoring for neurologic change using an objective quantifiable tool such as the NIHSS to alert clinicians to improvement or deterioration, warranting repeat of a STAT noncontrast CT to rule out sICH. Sudden onset of neurologic deterioration in the first 24 hours from treatment with IV-tPA is associated with either sICH or arterial reocclusion, which may occur in up to 22% of patients.[54] By closely assessing patients for neurologic change, reocclusion can be immediately identified and in some cases acted on by means of intra-arterial rescue.[3] Lastly, nurses and other interdisciplinary providers involved in the care of patients treated with IV-tPA must remember that once the drug has been administered, no invasive procedures may be performed for the next 24 hours unless there is a life-threatening need _and_ only when the invasive procedure is being performed on a compressible site.

For ischemic stroke patients with arterial occlusions evident on neuroimaging that may be treated within 8 hours of symptom onset, use of intra-arterial rescue procedures that include clot extraction using devices such as the MERCI retriever or Penumbra, angioplasty, or intra- and extracranial stent placement may be an option.[3] Often these treatment strategies are combined to ensure both clot clearance and vessel patency. Arterial access is typically achieved through canalization of the femoral artery. Serial angiograms are taken to diagnose the problem, strategize the treatment approach, and once treatment is complete, to evaluate the outcome. Patients undergoing intra-arterial treatment may require intubation and sedation, depending on the procedure undertaken and the preference of the interventionalist. Once the procedure is concluded, patients are often transported directly to MRI so that final infarct size can be determined. Nursing care of patients undergoing intra-arterial rescue procedures includes airway management, weaning and extubation, close monitoring and control of blood pressure before, during, and after the procedure, management of intraprocedural sedation, assessment of the groin arterial puncture site or maintenance of arterial sheaths when left in place, and ongoing neurologic monitoring using a quantifiable tool such as the NIHSS to determine change from baseline scores.

Malignant Ischemic Stroke

Sometimes, the even best reperfusion efforts fail, resulting in infarction. In patients with large infarctions affecting the cerebral hemispheres, and in particular the rare, young patient with a proximal middle cerebral artery occlusion that lacks room within the cranial vault that is typically associated with atrophic age-related changes, hemicraniectomy may be considered as a life-saving technique when intracranial mass effect with the risk of herniation is a concern.[55] Craniectomy may also be employed to treat cerebellar infarctions that risk compromise of brainstem structures due to edema and obstructive hydrocephalus.

Cautious patient selection and early timing before clinical deterioration are important considerations associated with optimal patient outcome. Practitioners should consider each patient individually for this lifesaving procedure, instead of automatically ruling out surgical intervention based on location of the lesion (ie, dominant hemispheric lesions), as many patients respond well regardless of the hemisphere implicated.[55]

Before surgery and during the postoperative phase of management, patients are managed for increased ICP, including such components as head of bed elevation to 30° with straight neck alignment, hypertonic saline or mannitol infusion, as well as intubation with sedation and analgesia. Intraventricular catheters are not employed in hemicraniectomy because of the significant brain displacement through the generous surgical defect that resolves compartmentalized pressure elevations. In craniectomy for cerebellar infarction, intraventricular drainage is employed, and is most commonly inserted after creation of the surgical defect to prevent a potential "upward" brain displacement with sudden reduction of ICP.

Postprocedural serial assessments using the NIHSS are important after hemicraniectomy and should be accompanied by noncontrast CT to determine response to therapy. Bone removed during hemicraniectomy procedures may be either stored in a Bone Bank or sewn into a pouch made in the patient's abdomen; the bone is replaced at around 3 months from the time of the brain infarction, and until that time clinicians may recommend that helmet precautions be followed when mobile.

EMERGING THERAPIES FOR HYPERACUTE ISCHEMIC STROKE
Sonothrombolysis

Concurrent treatment with IV-tPA and 2-mHz TCD insonation aimed at the arterial occlusion has been shown to be safe and efficacious for early neurologic improvement in a phase 2 randomized, placebo-controlled trial.[54] In sonothrombolysis, the approved full dose of IV-tPA is given using the methods previously described, and the TCD probe is fixated with a head frame so that the angle of insonation remains constant at the site of occlusion.[56] Compared with IV-tPA treatment alone, combined treatment with IV-tPA and 2-mHz TCD doubles the chance of arterial recanalization at 1 hour, and triples the chance of recanalization at 2 hours from the time of tPA bolus.[54] Limitations to the routine use of sonothrombolysis are primarily driven by the lack of physicians and technicians in North America capable of validly and reliably performing this technique. Current work is underway to develop a 2-mHz "hands-free" Doppler device that will automatically identify flow signal aberrancies and lock itself in the angle necessary to perform sonothrombolysis.

Induced Hypertension

Flow of blood through vessels is primarily determined by 2 factors: (1) Differences in pressure ($p_1 - p_2$) between the 2 ends of a vessel; and (2) vascular resistance to flow.[57,58] Ohm's law is often used to describe flow through the vascular system; simply put it states that blood flow is directly proportional to the pressure difference, but inversely proportional to the resistance[58]:

Blood flow $=$ Δpressure $\div$ resistance

It is theoretically sound to suggest that induced hypertension should increase blood flow through both partially occluded arteries and collateral vessels in patients with acute ischemic stroke, in that it drives the pressure component of the Ohm equation by increasing proximal p_1 pressures substantially over distal p_2 recipient vessels. Despite the clear theoretical-base supporting this practice, the literature is dominated by case reports, animal experiments, and only a few small human studies that have attempted to understand the effect of induced hypertension on neurologic outcome.

The widespread applicability of induced hypertension treatment is improbable; instead the need for this therapy is likely driven by specific occlusive lesion characteristics or central hemodynamic performance causing clinical fluctuation and deterioration. Because of this, it is unlikely that large clinical trials could be conceived, making induced hypertension an intervention with sound scientific underpinnings that is in a large way supported by the art of individualized hemodynamic augmentation.

Between 18% and 25% of acute ischemic stroke patients present with arterial blood pressures less than 140 mm Hg systolic.[59,60] Thirty-day mortality is significantly higher in patients with lower blood pressure, and is probably related to several contributing factors including reduced perfusion to ischemic brain tissue and concurrent myocardial dysfunction. The primary cause of low blood pressure in the early stages of stroke has been primarily associated with preexisting known or occult heart disease, although other causes including sepsis, hypovolemia, and centrally mediated reflexes that support myocardial and vasomotor function may also be implicated.

Because there is no consistent definition of the "best" baseline hemodynamic and clinical parameters that would indicate suitability for induced hypertension therapy,[59,61] patient selection is largely dependent on practitioners' individualized assessment of systemic and stroke territory vascular dynamics in concert with clinical presentation. The literature identifies several agents that have been used for induced hypertension, including phenylephrine, norepinephrine, epinephrine, and dopamine.[62–75] Of these, phenylephrine is by far the most common agent represented in published studies, most likely due to its selective α1-adrenergic effects that constrict the peripheral vasculature without producing constriction in the brain's arterial circuit.[62]

In the case of suboptimal myocardial contractility, application of an α1-adrenergic agent such as phenylephrine becomes more complex, in that although capable of increasing central arterial pressures, cardiac output may actually decrease due to increased left ventricular afterload. In this scenario, use of an inotrope with minimal chronotropic effects such as dobutamine should be considered alongside delivery of phenylephrine.

Induced Hypervolemic Therapy

Theoretical support for induced hypervolemia is based on the potential for increased blood viscosity in ischemic stroke due to increased fibrinogen levels, red cell aggregation, and leukocyte activation, with a presumed ability to increase collateral blood flow with volume treatment.[76] Hypervolemic therapy alone has not been fully evaluated. Instead, hypervolemia was combined with hemodilution (HHD) to more thoroughly reduce blood viscosity in several studies in the late 1980s to 1990s, to evaluate whether this would benefit neurologic outcome in patients with acute stroke.[76–83] Of importance is that individualized assessment of intravascular volume in relation to myocardial contractility in accordance with Frank-Starling was not included in these studies, so one is unable to conclude just how optimal or suboptimal was the ventricular stretch that resulted from these treatments.

Methods reported in the literature for achieving HHD include a combination of venesection and replacement of the same volume of blood removed with either dextran 40 in saline solution[77–79] or 10% hydroxyethyl starch 200/0.5[80,81]; treatment in these studies was continued for 5 to 7 days. Two smaller trials identified improvement in patients receiving HHD,[81,82] whereas larger trials failed to find benefit associated with HHD treatment in acute stroke.[76–80] A modest number of patients in these studies developed complications associated with pulmonary edema secondary to congestive heart failure. A Cochrane review, which includes 3119 patients in 18 clinical trials using HHD in acute stroke, found no benefit from incorporation of this therapy on 4-week mortality, 3- to 6-month mortality, and 3- to 6-month death/dependency rates.[76] What remains unknown is whether hypervolemic therapy delivered to a point of optimal ventricular stretch, in combination with induced hypertension supported by inotropic dobutamine therapy, may benefit perfusion and clinical outcome in acute stroke patients. Only one small study reports using these methods which, while more complex, are more likely to maintain physiologic balance between the cardiac and systemic hemodynamic circuits.[83]

More recently, interest has shifted to the neuroprotective effects of 25% albumin given in amounts that may constitute hypervolemic therapy through both direct volume administration and extravascular-to-intravascular fluid shifts.[84] Human serum albumin is a potent antioxidant with neuroprotective findings that include improved neurologic scores, decreased infarction volume, reduced brain swelling, decreased metabolism-blood flow dissociation in injured brain, improved cerebral perfusion, diffusion image normalization, and reversal of microvascular stasis.[84–91]

The ongoing ALIAS (Albumin in Acute Stroke) clinical trial is investigating the use of a 2 g/kg infusion of human serum albumin in acute ischemic stroke as a neuroprotective agent given within 5 hours of symptom onset. The primary end point is achievement of an NIH stroke scale score of 0 to 1 or a modified Rankin scale score of 0 to 1 at 3 months; the safety end point is incidence of congestive heart failure after study-drug administration.[92] The study consists of two 900-subject cohorts, one with and one without treatment with intravenous tPA by standard of care criteria.[93]

Pilot work in support of ALIAS included enrollment of 82 subjects (mean age 65 years; NIHSS scores 6 or greater) who received a 25% albumin infusion within 16 hours of stroke onset (7.8 ± 3.4 hours); an additional 42 patients were also treated with intravenous tPA. Six successive dose tiers were assessed (range, 0.34–2.05 g/kg). Maximum increases in plasma albumin and mild hemodilution were apparent at 4 to 12 hours into treatment. Plasma brain natriuretic peptide levels increased at 24 hours but did not predict cardiac adverse events, and mild to moderate pulmonary edema amenable to diuretic therapy occurred in 13.4% of subjects. One subject (2.4%) in the tPA-treated group developed symptomatic intracerebral hemorrhage.[94] At 3 months, the highest 3 therapeutic dose tiers (1.37–2.05 g/kg) were compared with the lowest 3 doses that were presumed to be subtherapeutic (0.34–1.03 g/kg). The probability of achieving a modified Rankin Scale 0 to 1 or NIHSS 0 to 1 at 3 months among subjects in the highest 3 dose tiers was 81% greater than in subjects in the lower dose tiers (relative risk [RR] = 1.81; 95% confidence interval [CI] = 1.11–2.94), and was 95% greater than the NINDS rt-PA Stroke Study placebo cohort (RR = 1.95; 95% CI = 1.47–2.57). Subjects treated with tPA who received the higher albumin dose were 3 times more likely to achieve the end point than subjects in lower dose tiers, which the investigators conclude may indicate a positive synergistic effect between tPA and human serum albumin treatment.[95]

Although it remains to be seen what the ultimate effect of human albumin treatment will be in acute ischemic stroke, prudent use of any therapy that has the potential to increase intravascular volume must be considered alongside each subject's inherent myocardial function. Without such cautious consideration, the potential neuroprotective effects of this agent may be overshadowed by deleterious cardiovascular outcomes, rendering a potentially beneficial treatment as a failure in reducing disability associated with stroke.

Correction of Reversed Robin Hood Syndrome

The prevalence of sleep apnea in stroke patients ranges from 30% to 70%.[96,97] It remains unclear how often sleep apnea in stroke patients is of central, obstructive, or mixed etiologies, and although all patients suspected for this disorder should receive formal sleep studies, the early identification and management of sleep-associated disordered breathing should be promptly undertaken by stroke practitioners. The "Reversed Robin Hood syndrome" (RRHS) documents intravascular "steal" of blood from neurovascular territories associated with stroke that need optimal perfusion, to normal vascular territories during apneic episodes.[98]

The pathophysiology supporting RRHS suggests that vasomotor reactivity in response to elevated carbon dioxide levels is lost in the arterial region of the stroke due to ischemia, which depletes cellular adenosine triphosphate stores, although vasomotor reactivity is maintained in normally perfused areas of the brain; during apneic episodes with elevated arterial carbon dioxide levels, normal vasculature in the brain vasodilates, thereby "stealing" arterial blood flow away from ischemic regions that are unable to dilate in response to carbon dioxide levels. Quantifiable clinical worsening has been noted in response to RRHS due to increased penumbral ischemia.[98] Use of noninvasive modes of ventilation with continuous positive airway pressure have been shown to improve and maintain steady arterial flow through neurovascular territories in patients with sleep apnea, while improving and maintaining clinical outcome.[96] Nurses working with stroke patients will increasingly need to become expert in the use of noninvasive ventilation, as its use will continue to grow in the coming years to combat sleep-disordered breathing problems such as apnea.

Mechanical Devices for Hemodynamic Augmentation

External counterpulsation

Noninvasive external counterpulsation (ECP) was approved in the United States in the 1990s for use in patients with multivessel coronary artery disease, refractory angina pectoris, acute myocardial infarction with cardiogenic shock, and most recently congestive heart failure.[99–102] As with an intra-aortic balloon pump (IABP), ECP is triggered by electrocardiography, which causes pressure application (300 mm Hg) during diastole that is delivered by air-filled cuffs placed around the lower abdomen/buttocks and legs **(Fig. 4)**.[99,100]

The hemodynamic effects of ECP have been shown to be equivalent to IABP,[103,104] with cuff inflation causing increased coronary, brain,[105–108] eye, and upper extremity perfusion, and the sudden cuff deflation before systole resulting in improved lower extremity and renal perfusion as well as decreased resistance to outflow from the left ventricle.[104,109–118] The effects of ECP also include development and recruitment of collateral vessels in ischemic territories,[119–121] and Windkessel effect enhancement has been tied to an increase in nitric oxide expression due to increased arterial wall stress during ECP cuff inflation.[122] ECP effects on vascular endothelial cell morphology demonstrate a reduction of cellular adherence to cholesterol-rich plaques with improved endothelial cell parallel alignment with blood flow, and a significant decrease in intimal hyperplasia following serial treatments.[122]

In normal controls, ECP produces an almost 200% increase in diastolic flow velocities on transcranial Doppler during device inflation, with an overall mean flow velocity increase in normal subjects of 120% on average.[123] In subacute ischemic stroke patients, ECP has been shown to be safe and capable of reducing neurologic disability on the NIHSS when used as distant as 7 to 14 weeks from stroke onset.[124]

At present, the "dose" of ECP that may be useful in acute stroke patients remains unknown, and application of the cardiac dose (35 daily, 1-hour treatments delivered as 5 treatments a week for 7 weeks) in acute ischemic stroke patients is likely to be

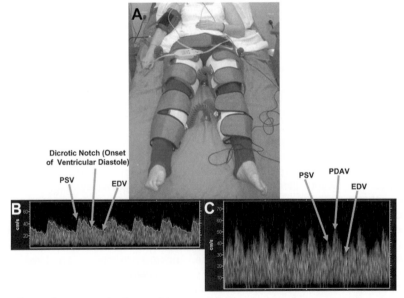

Fig. 4. External counterpulsation and transcranial Doppler waveforms.

unfeasible due to short hospital stays in many countries and the need for daily transport to receive ECP treatment once discharged. Work exploring methods to dose ECP in acute ischemic stroke patients who are not candidates for reperfusion therapy is ongoing at present.

A second limitation of the device is related to the cuff inflation sequences. During cuff inflation, the lower torso is thrust upward in a somewhat violent manner and then released during deflation, with this repeated in time with the cardiac cycle. Given a normal heart rate the device would inflate and then deflate in this manner approximately 80 to 100 times per minute over a period of 1 hour. This repetitive rate limits the use of the device in patients with invasive technology that is sensitive to disruption (ie, endotracheal tubes, ventriculostomies). It also limits use of ECP in patients with back injuries, which may become aggravated due to rhythmic movement.

Partial aortic occlusion

The NeuroFlo catheter emerged in the 1990s as a simple intra-aortic device capable of producing improved cerebral blood flow (CBF) through a single, 45-minute inflation.[125,126] While approved by the Food and Drug Administration for use in aneurysmal subarachnoid hemorrhage with vasospasm, the device continues to undergo evaluation for use in ischemic stroke. Preliminary data suggest an ability of the catheter to improve periprocedural cerebral perfusion markers and reduce neurologic impairment on NIHSS, both in the periprocedural phase and at 24 hours posttreatment.[126] The NeuroFlo carries a similar limitation to IABP in that it is invasive. In addition, other than data reported in a swine stroke model, impact of the device on left ventricular afterload due to continuous balloon inflation throughout the cardiac cycle remains unknown, although it is considered unsuitable for use in patients with concurrent cardiac dysfunction.

The NeuroFlo catheter is inserted in the catheterization laboratory, and balloons are inflated for only a 45-minute period. Following balloon deflation, the device is removed. Despite its short inflation period, it has been shown to have sustained effects on CBF, most likely through a combination of direct transluminal residual blood flow coupled with recruitment of collateral channels that would have remained otherwise dormant, and perhaps even venous retrograde flow. Several ongoing stroke studies are underway to evaluate the use of this less complex therapy in acute ischemic stroke, including persistence of any hemodynamic and clinical effect arising from this therapy.

SUMMARY

Hyperacute ischemic stroke management requires a commitment to discovery and delivery of aggressive front-line therapies. Today's most progressive acute stroke practitioners find reasons "to treat" patients, instead of identifying reasons "to withhold treatment." Hyperacute stroke science is driven by an inquisitive interest in intracranial and systemic hemodynamic therapies, coupled with a determination to reverse neurologic dysfunction. Nurses practicing in this area are challenged to expand their expertise to incorporate the assessment and management of altered vascular dynamics, while embracing a shift in the stroke treatment paradigm toward pursuit of improved methods to reduce neurologic disability and death.

REFERENCES

1. Kidwell CS, Starkman S, Eckstein M, et al. Identifying stroke in the field: prospective validation of the Los Angeles Prehospital Stroke Screen (LAPSS). Stroke 2000;31:71–6.

2. Kothari RU, Pancioli A, Liu T, et al. Cincinnati prehospital stroke scale: reproducibility and validity. Ann Emerg Med 1999;33:373–8.
3. Adams HP, del Zoppo G, Alberts MJ, et al. Guidelines for the early management of adults with ischemic stroke. Stroke 2007;38:1655–711.
4. Suyama J, Crocco T. Prehospital care of the stroke patient. Emerg Med Clin North Am 2002;20:537–52.
5. Silliman SL, Quinn B, Hugget V, et al. Use of a field-to-stroke center helicopter transport program to extend thrombolytic therapy to rural residents. Stroke 2003;34:729–33.
6. Rymer MM, Thrutchley DE, Stroke Team at the Mid America Brain and Stroke Institute. Organizing regional networks to increase acute stroke intervention. Neurol Res 2005;27(Suppl 1):S9–16.
7. Rossnagel K, Jungehusing GJ, Nolte CH, et al. Out-of-hospital delays in patients with acute stroke. Ann Emerg Med 2004;44:476–83.
8. Porteous GH, Corry MD, Smith WS. Emergency medical services dispatcher identification of stroke and transient ischemic attack. Prehosp Emerg Care 1999;3:211–6.
9. Morris DL, Rosamond W, Madden K, et al. Prehospital and emergency department delays after acute stroke: the Genentech Stroke Presentation Survey. Stroke 2000;31:2585–90.
10. Williams JE, Rosamond WD, Morris DL. Stroke symptom attribution and time to emergency department arrival: the delay in accessing stroke healthcare study. Acad Emerg Med 2000;7:93–6.
11. Schroeder EB, Rosamond WD, Morris DL, et al. Determinants of use of emergency medical services in a population with stroke symptoms: the Second Delay in Accessing Stroke Healthcare (DASH II) Study. Stroke 2000;31:2591–6.
12. Lacy CR, Suh DC, Bueno M, et al. Delay in presentation and evaluation for acute stroke: Stroke Time Registry for Outcomes Knowledge and Epidemiology (S.T.R.O.K.E.). Stroke 2001;32:63–9.
13. Wojner-Alexandrov AW, Alexandrov AV, Rodriguez D, et al. Houston paramedic and emergency stroke treatment and outcomes study (HoPSTO). Stroke 2005;36:1512–8.
14. Schwamm LH, Pancioli A, Acker JE 3rd, et al. American Stroke Association's Task Force on the Development of Stroke Systems. Recommendations for the establishment of stroke systems of care: recommendations from the American Stroke Association's Task Force on the Development of Stroke Systems. Stroke 2005;36:690–703.
15. Tanabe P, Travers D, Gilboy N, et al. Refining emergency severity index triage criteria. Acad Emerg Med 2005;12(6):497–501.
16. Tanabe P, Gimbel R, Yarnold PR, et al. Reliability and validity of scores on The Emergency Severity Index version 3. Acad Emerg Med 2004;11(1):59–65.
17. NINDS Proceedings of a National Symposium on Rapid Identification and Treatment of Acute Stroke. Available at: http://www.ninds.nih.gov/news_and_events/proceedings/stroke_proceedings/recs-emerg.htm. 1996. Accessed June 17, 2009.
18. Alberts MJ, Hademenos G, Latchaw RE, et al. Brain Attack Coalition. Recommendations for the establishment of primary stroke centers. JAMA 2000;283:3102–9.
19. Alberts MJ, Latchaw RE, Selman WR, et al. Brain Attack Coalition. Recommendations for comprehensive stroke centers: a consensus statement from the Brain Attack Coalition. Stroke 2005;36:1597–616.

20. Grotta JC, Chiu D, Lu M, et al. Agreement and variability in the interpretation of early CT changes in stroke patients qualifying for intravenous rtPA therapy. Stroke 1999;30:1528–33.
21. Kidwell CS, Chalela JA, Saver JL, et al. Comparison of MRI and CT for detection of acute intracerebral hemorrhage. JAMA 2004;292:1823–30.
22. Patel SC, Levine SR, Tilley BC, et al. National Institute of Neurological Disorders and Stroke rt-PA Stroke Study Group. Lack of clinical significance of early ischemic changes on computed tomography in acute stroke. JAMA 2001;286:2830–8.
23. Kasner SE. Clinical interpretation and use of stroke scales. Lancet Neurol 2006;5(7):603–12.
24. Dominguez R, Vila JF, Augustovski F, et al. Spanish cross-cultural adaption and validation of the National Institutes of Health Stroke Scale. Mayo Clin Proc 2006;81(4):476–80.
25. Lyden P, Lu M, Jackson C, et al. Underlying structure of the National Institutes of Health Stroke Scale: results of a factor analysis. NINDS tPA Stroke Trial Investigators. Stroke 1999;30(11):2347–54.
26. Dewey HM, Donnan GA, Freeman EJ, et al. Interrater reliability of the National Institutes of Health Stroke Scale: Rating by neurologists and nurses in a community-based stroke incidence study. Cerebrovasc Dis 1999;9(6):323–7.
27. Lyden P, Brott T, Tilley B, et al. Improved reliability of the NIH Stroke Scale using video training. NINDS TPA Stroke Study Group. Stroke 1994;25(11):2220–6.
28. Goldstein LB, Samsa GP. Reliability of the National Institutes of Health Stroke Scale: extension to non-neurologists in the context of a clinical trial. Stroke 1997;28:307–10.
29. Lyden P, Raman R, Liu L, et al. NIHSS training and certification using a new digital video disk is reliable. Stroke 2005;36(11):2446–9.
30. Josephson SA, Hills NK, Johnston SC. NIH Stroke Scale reliability in ratings from a large sample of clinicians. Cerebrovasc Dis 2006;22(5–6):389–95.
31. Wojner-Alexandrov AW, Garami Z, Chernyshev OY, et al. Heads down: Flat head positioning improves blood flow velocities in acute ischemic stroke. Neurology 2005;64(8):1354–7.
32. Hacke W, Kaste M, Bluhmki E, et al. ECASS Investigators. Thrombolysis with Alteplase 3 to 4.5 hours after acute ischemic stroke. N Engl J Med 2008;59(13):1317–29.
33. The National Institute of Neurological Disorders and Stroke rt-PA Stroke Study Group. Tissue plasminogen activator for acute ischemic stroke. N Engl J Med 1995;333(24):1581–7.
34. Albers GW, Bates VE, Clark WM, et al. Intravenous tissue-type plasminogen activator for treatment of acute stroke: the Standard Treatment with Alteplase to Reverse Stroke (STARS) study. JAMA 2000;283(9):1145–50.
35. Hill MD, Buchan AM. Canadian Alteplase for Stroke Effectiveness Study (CASES) Investigators. Thrombolysis for acute ischemic stroke: results of the Canadian Alteplase for Stroke Effectiveness Study. CMAJ 2005;172(10):1307–12.
36. Steiner T, Bluhmki E, Kaste M, et al. The ECASS 3-hour cohort. Secondary analysis of ECASS data by time stratification. ECASS Study Group. European Cooperative Acute Stroke Study. Cerebrovasc Dis 1998;8(4):198–203.
37. Hacke W, Kaste M, Fieschi C, et al. Randomised double-blind placebo-controlled trial of thrombolytic therapy with intravenous alteplase in acute ischaemic stroke (ECASS II). Second European-Australasian Acute Stroke Study Investigators. Lancet 1998;352(9136):1245–51.

38. Hacke W, Donnan G, Fieschi C, et al. ATLANTIS Trials Investigators; ECASS Trials Investigators; NINDS rt-PA Study Group Investigators. Association of outcome with early stroke treatment: pooled analysis of ATLANTIS, ECASS, and NINDS rt-PA stroke trials. Lancet 2004;363(9411):768–74.

39. Wahlgren N, Ahmed N, Davalos A, et al. For the SITS-MOST Investigators. Thrombolysis with alteplase for acute ischaemic stroke in the safe implementation of thrombolysis in stroke-monitoring study (SITS-MOST): an observational study. Lancet 2007;369(9558):275–82.

40. Castillo J, Leira R, Garcia MM, et al. Blood pressure decrease during the acute phase of ischemic stroke is associated with brain injury and poor stroke outcome. Stroke 2004;35:520–6.

41. Johnston KC, Mayer SA. Blood pressure reduction in ischemic stroke: a two-edged sword? Neurology 2003;61:1030–1.

42. Williams LS, Rotich J, Qi R, et al. Effects of admission hyperglycemia on mortality and costs in acute ischemic stroke. Neurology 2002;59:67–71.

43. Scott JF, Robinson GM, French JM, et al. Prevalence of admission hyperglycaemia across clinical subtypes of acute stroke. Lancet 1999;353:376–7.

44. Baird TA, Parsons MW, Barber PA, et al. The influence of diabetes mellitus and hyperglycaemia on stroke incidence and outcome. J Clin Neurosci 2002;9:618–26.

45. Gray CS, Hildreth AJ, Alberti GK, et al. GIST Collaboration. Poststroke hyperglycemia: natural history and immediate management. Stroke 2004;35:122–6.

46. Azzimondi G, Bassein L, Nonino F, et al. Fever in acute stroke worsens prognosis: a prospective study. Stroke 1995;26:2040–3.

47. Reith J, Jorgensen HS, Pedersen PM, et al. Body temperature in acute stroke: relation to stroke severity, infarct size, mortality, and outcome. Lancet 1996; 347:422–5.

48. Castillo J, Davalos A, Marrugat J, et al. Timing for fever-related brain damage in acute ischemic stroke. Stroke 1998;29:2455–60.

49. Ginsberg MD, Busto R. Combating hyperthermia in acute stroke: a significant clinical concern. Stroke 1998;29:529–34.

50. Hajat C, Hajat S, Sharma P. Effects of poststroke pyrexia on stroke outcome: a meta-analysis of studies in patients. Stroke 2000;31:410–4.

51. Wang Y, Lim LL, Levi C, et al. Influence of admission body temperature on stroke mortality. Stroke 2000;31:404–9.

52. Kammersgaard LP, Jorgensen HS, Rungby JA, et al. Admission body temperature predicts long-term mortality after acute stroke: the Copenhagen Stroke Study. Stroke 2002;33:1759–62.

53. Zaremba J. Hyperthermia in ischemic stroke. Med Sci Monit 2004;10:RA148–53.

54. Alexandrov AV, Molina CA, Grotta JC, et al. CLOTBUST Investigators. Ultrasound-enhanced systemic thrombolysis for acute ischemic stroke. N Engl J Med 2004;351(21):2170–8.

55. Vahedi K, Hofmeijer J, Juettler E, et al. DECIMAL, DESTINY, and HAMLET investigators. Early decompressive surgery in malignant middle cerebral artery infarction: pooled analysis of three randomized controlled trials. Lancet Neurol 2007;6:215–22.

56. Alexandrov AV, Wojner AW, Grotta JC, CLOTBUST investigators. CLOTBUST: Design of a randomized trial of ultrasound-enhanced thrombolysis for acute stroke. J Neuroimaging 2004;14:108–12.

57. Alexandrov AW. Integrated systemic and intracranial hemodynamics. In: Alexandrov AV, editor. Cerebrovascular ultrasound in stroke prevention and treatment. Armonk (NY): Blackwell Futura; 2003. p. 41–61.

58. Guyton AC. Textbook of medical physiology. 11th edition. Philadelphia: W.B. Saunders; 2005.
59. International Stroke Trial Collaborative Group. The International StrokeTrial (IST): a randomised trial of aspirin, subcutaneous heparin, both, or neither among 19 435 patients with acute ischaemic stroke. Lancet 1997;349:1569–81.
60. Mistri AK, Robinson TG, Potter JF. Pressor therapy in acute ischemic stroke: systematic review. Stroke 2006;37:1565–71.
61. Blood pressure in Acute Stroke Collaboration (BASC). Interventions for deliberately altering blood pressure in acute stroke. Cochrane Database Syst Rev 2001;(2):CD000039. DOI:10.1002/14651858.
62. Ishikawa S, Ito H, Yokoyama K, et al. Phenylephrine ameliorates cerebral cytotoxic edema and reduces cerebral infarction volume in a rat model of complete unilateral carotid artery occlusion with severe hypotension. Anesth Analg 2008; 108(5):1631–7.
63. Stead LG, Bellolio MF, Gilmore RM, et al. Pharmacologic elevation of blood pressure for acute brain ischemia. Neurocrit Care 2008;8(2):259–61.
64. Shin HK, Nishimura M, Jones PB, et al. Mild induced hypertension improves blood flow and oxygen metabolism in transient focal cerebral ischemia. Stroke 2008;39(5):1548–55.
65. Kim HF, Kang DW. Induced hypertensive therapy in an acute ischemic stroke patient with early neurological deterioration. J Clin Neurol 2007;3(4):187–91.
66. Bogoslovsky T, Happola O, Salonen O, et al. Induced hypertension for the treatment of acute MCA occlusion beyond the thrombolysis window: case report. BMC Neurol 2006;19(6):46.
67. Rose JC, Mayer SA. Optimizing blood pressure in neurological emergencies. Neurocrit Care 2004;1(3):287–99.
68. Marzan AS, Hungerbuhler HJ, Studer A, et al. Feasibility and safety of norepinephrine-induced arterial hypertension in acute ischemic stroke. Neurology 2004;62(7):1193–5.
69. Hillis AE, Ulatowski JA, Barker PB, et al. A pilot randomized trial of induced blood pressure elevation: effects on function and focal perfusion in acute and subacute stroke. Cerebrovasc Dis 2003;16(3):236–46.
70. Schwarz S, Georgiadis D, Aschoff A, et al. Effects of induced hypertension on intracranial pressure and flow velocities of the middle cerebral arteries in patients with large hemispheric stroke. Stroke 2002;33(4):998–1004.
71. Oliverira-Filho J, Pedreira BB, Jesus PA, et al. Pharmacologically-induced hypertension in a patient with vertebro-basilar territory ischemia associated with bilateral vertebral stenosis. Arq Neuropsiquiatr 2002;60(2-B):498–501.
72. Hillis AE, Kane A, Tuffiash E, et al. Reperfusion of specific brain regions by raising blood pressure restores selective language functions in subacute stroke. Brain Lang 2001;79(3):495–510.
73. Rordorf G, Cramer SC, Efird JT, et al. Pharmacological elevation of blood pressure in acute stroke. Clinical effects and safety. Stroke 1997;28(11): 21133–2138.
74. Drummond JC, Oh YS, Cole DJ, et al. Phenylephrine-induced hypertension reduces ischemia following middle cerebral artery occlusion in rats. Stroke 1989;20(11):1538–44.
75. Hayashi S, Nehls DG, Kieck CF, et al. Beneficial effects of induced hypertension on experimental stroke in awake monkeys. J Neurosurg 1984;60(1):151–7.
76. Asplund K. Haemodilution for acute ischaemic stroke. Cochrane Database Syst Rev 2002;(4):CD000103. DOI:10.1002/14651858.

77. Multicenter trial of hemodilution in acute ischemic stroke. I. Results in the total patient population. Scandinavian Stroke Study Group. Stroke 1987;18(4):691–9.

78. Multicenter trial of hemodilution in acute ischemic stroke. Results of subgroup analyses. Scandinavian Stroke Study Group. Stroke 1988;19(4):464–71.

79. Italian Acute Stroke Study Group. Haemodilution in acute stroke: results of the Italian haemodilution trial. Lancet 1988;1(8581):318–21.

80. Aichner FT, Fazekas F, Brainin M, et al. Hypervolemic hemodilution in acute ischemic stroke: the Multicenter Austrian Hemodilution Stroke Trial (MAHST). Stroke 1998;29:743–9.

81. Hypervolemic hemodilution treatment of acute stroke. Results of a randomized multicenter trial using pentastarch. The Hemodilution in Stroke Study Group. Stroke 1989;20(3):317–23.

82. Strand T. Evaluation of long-term outcome and safety after hemodilution therapy in acute ischemic stroke. Stroke 1992;23(5):657–62.

83. Duke BJ, Breeze RE, Rubenstein D, et al. Induced hypervolemia and inotropic support for acute cerebral arterial insufficiency: an underused therapy. Surg Neurol 1998;49(1):51–4.

84. Belayev L, Liu Y, Zhao W, et al. Human albumin therapy of acute ischemic stroke: marked neuroprotective efficacy at moderate doses and with a broad therapeutic window. Stroke 2001;32:553–60.

85. Gum ET, Swanson RA, Alano C, et al. Human serum albumin and its N-terminal tetrapeptide (DAHK) block oxidant-induced neuronal death. Stroke 2004;35(2): 590–5.

86. Belayev L, Alonso OF, Busto R, et al. Middle cerebral artery occlusion in the rat by intraluminal suture. Neurological and pathological evaluation of an improved model. Stroke 1996;27:1616–22.

87. Belayev L, Busto R, Zhao W, et al. Effect of delayed albumin hemodilution on infarction volume and brain edema after transient middle cerebral artery occlusion in rats. J Neurosurg 1997;87:595–601.

88. Belayev L, Zhao W, Pattany PM, et al. Diffusion-weighted magnetic resonance imaging confirms marked neuroprotective efficacy of albumin therapy in focal cerebral ischemia. Stroke 1998;29:2587–99.

89. Liu Y, Belayev L, Zhao W, et al. Neuroprotective effect of treatment with human albumin in permanent focal cerebral ischemia: histopathology and cortical perfusion studies. Eur J Pharmacol 2001;428:193–201.

90. Ginsberg MD, Zhao W, Belayev L, et al. Diminution of metabolism/blood flow uncoupling following traumatic brain injury in rats in response to high-dose human albumin treatment. J Neurosurg 2001;94(3):499–509.

91. Belayev L, Marcheselli VL, Khoutorova L, et al. Docosahexaenoic acid complexed to albumin elicits high-grade ischemic neuroprotection. Stroke 2005;36(1):118–23.

92. Hill MD, Moy CS, Palesch YY, et al. ALIAS Investigators. The albumin in acute stroke trial (ALIAS); design and methodology. Int J Stroke 2007;2(3):214–9.

93. Ginsberg MD, Palesch YY, Hill MD. The ALIAS (ALbumin In Acute Stroke) Phase III randomized multicentre clinical trial: design and progress report. Biochem Soc Trans 2006;34(Pt 6):1323–6.

94. Ginsberg MD, Hill MD, Palesch YY, et al. The ALIAS Pilot Trial: a dose-escalation and safety study of albumin therapy for acute ischemic stroke—I: physiological responses and safety results. Stroke 2006;37(8):2100–6.

95. Palesch YY, Hill MD, Ryckborst KJ, et al. The ALIAS Pilot Trial: a dose-escalation and safety study of albumin therapy for acute ischemic stroke—II: neurologic outcome and efficacy analysis. Stroke 2006;37(8):2107–14.

96. Martinez-Garcia MA, Galiano-Blancart R, Roman-Sanchez P, et al. Continuous positive airway pressure treatment in sleep apnea prevents new vascular events after ischemic stroke. Chest 2005;128:2123–9.

97. Culebras A. Sleep apnea and stroke. Rev Neurol Dis 2005;2:13–9.

98. Alexandrov AV, Sharma VK, Lao AY, et al. Reversed Robin Hood syndrome in acute ischemic stroke patients. Stroke 2007;38(11):3045–8.

99. Werner D, Schneider M, Weise M, et al. Pneumatic external counterpulsation: a new noninvasive method to improve organ perfusion. Am J Cardiol 1999; 84(8):950–2, A7–8.

100. Arora RR, Chou TM, Jain D, et al. The multicenter study of enhanced external counterpulsation (MUST-EECP): effect of EECP on exercise-induced myocardial ischemia and anginal episodes. J Am Coll Cardiol 1999;33(7):1833–40.

101. Cohn PF. Enhanced external counterpulsation for the treatment of angina pectoris. Prog Cardiovasc Dis 2006;49(2):88–97.

102. Feldman AM, Silver MA, Francis GS, et al. PEECH Investigators. Enhanced external counterpulsation improves exercise tolerance in patients with chronic heart failure. J Am Coll Cardiol 2006;48(6):1198–205.

103. Taguchi I, Ogawa K, Oida A, et al. Comparison of hemodynamic effects of enhanced external counterpulsation and intra-aortic balloon pumping in patients with acute myocardial infarction. Am J Cardiol 2000;86(10):1139–41, A9.

104. Masuda D, Nohara R, Hirai T, et al. Enhanced external counterpulsation improved myocardial perfusion and coronary flow reserve in patients with chronic stable angina. Eur Heart J 2001;22:1451–8.

105. Applebaum RM, Kasliwal R, Tunick PA, et al. Sequential external counterpulsation increases cerebral and renal blood flow. Am Heart J 1997;133:611–5.

106. Kern MJ, Aguirre FV, Caracciola EA, et al. Hemodynamic effects of new intra-aortic balloon counterpulsation timing methods in patients: a multicenter evaluation. Am Heart J 1999;137(6):1129–36.

107. Werner D, Marthol H, Brown CM, et al. Changes of cerebral blood flow velocities during enhanced external counterpulsation. Acta Neurol Scand 2003;107: 405–11.

108. Marthol H, Werner D, Brown CM, et al. Enhanced external counterpulsation does not compromise cerebral autoregulation. Acta Neurol Scand 2005;111:34–41.

109. Hilz MJ, Werner D, Marthol H, et al. Enhanced external counterpulsation improves skin oxygenation and perfusion. Eur J Clin Invest 2004;34(6):385–91.

110. Levenson J, Simon A, Megnien JL, et al. Effects of enhanced external counterpulsation on carotid circulation in patients with coronary artery disease. Cardiology 2006;108:104–10.

111. Werner D, Michelson G, Harazny J, et al. Changes in ocular blood flow velocities during external counterpulsation in healthy volunteers and patients with atherosclerosis. Graefes Arch Clin Exp Ophthalmol 2001;239(8):599–602.

112. Werner D, Michalk F, Harazny J, et al. Accelerated reperfusion of poorly perfused retinal areas in central retinal artery occlusion and branch retinal artery occlusion after a short treatment with enhanced external counterpulsation. Retina 2004;24(4):541–7.

113. Werner D, Tragner P, Wawer A, et al. Enhanced external counterpulsation: a new technique to augment renal function in liver cirrhosis. Nephrol Dial Transplant 2005;20(5):920–6.

114. Michaels AD, Accad M, Ports TA, et al. Left ventricular systolic unloading and augmentation of intracoronary pressure and Doppler flow during enhanced external counterpulsation. Circulation 2002;106(10):1237–42.

115. Michaels AD, Linnemeier G, Soran O, et al. Two-year outcomes after enhanced external counterpulsation for stable angina pectoris from the International EECP Patient Registry (IEPR). Am J Cardiol 2004;93(4):461–4.
116. Fitzgerald CP, Lawson WE, Hui JC, et al. IEPR Investigators. Enhanced external counterpulsation as initial revascularization treatment for angina refractory to medical therapy. Cardiology 2003;100(3):129–35.
117. Yi Y, Yang Y, Jian C. Cerebral hemodynamic impairment and therapeutic effect of external counterpulsation on elderly patients with brain infarction. Hunan Yi Ke Da Xue Xue Bao 1999;24(5):435–7.
118. Yi YX, Zhu XP, Yang Y. Therapeutic hemodynamic effects of external counterpulsation on elderly patients with brain infarction during convalescence. Hunan Yi Ke Da Xue Xue Bao 2000;25(1):45–7.
119. Amsterdam EZ, Banas J, Criley JM, et al. Clinical assessment of external pressure circulatory assistance in acute myocardial infarction. Am J Cardiol 1980;45: 349–56.
120. Urano H, Ikeda H, Ueno T, et al. Enhanced external counterpulsation improves exercise tolerance, reduces exercise-induced myocardial ischemia and improves left ventricular diastolic filling in patients with coronary artery disease. J Am Coll Cardiol 2001;37(1):93–9.
121. Bagger JP, Hall RJ, Loutroulis G, et al. Effect of enhanced external counterpulsation on dobutamine-induced left ventricular wall motion abnormalities in severe chronic angina pectoris. Am J Cardiol 2004;93(4):465–7.
122. Zhang Y, He X, Chen X, et al. Enhanced external counterpulsation inhibits intimal hyperplasia by modifying shear stress-responsive gene expression in hypercholesterolemic pigs. Circulation 2007;116:526–34.
123. Alexandrov AW, Ribo M, Wong KS, et al. Perfusion augmentation in acute stroke using mechanical counterpulsation—(PUMP) Phase IIA. Effect of external counterpulsation (ECP) on middle cerebral artery mean flow velocity in five healthy subjects. Stroke 2008;39. Stroke ASAP (on-line ahead of print), July 24, 2008, 10.1161/STROKEAHA.107.512418.
124. Han J, Leung TW, Lam WW, et al. External counterpulsation for recent ischemic stroke patients with large artery occlusive disease. Stroke 2008;39(4):1340–3.
125. Barbut D. Effect of aortic occlusion on intracerebral blood flow in acute stroke. International Stroke Conference. Stroke 2003.
126. Shuaib A. The SENTIS trial: endovascular augmentation of collateral flow, 2007, International Stroke Conference, San Francisco (CA), February 16, 2007.

Migraine and Patent Foramen Ovale: State of the Science

CindyJ. Fuller, PhD, Jill T. Jesurum, PhD, ARNP, FAHA*

KEYWORDS

• Migraine • Headache • Patent foramen ovale • Stroke • Aura

An association between migraine and patent foramen ovale (PFO) has been noted in a number of investigations[1–6] and has led to speculation that microemboli and vasoactive chemicals transmitted through the PFO can trigger migraine symptoms in susceptible persons.[1] Interestingly, the only prospective, randomized trial to evaluate the effects of transcatheter PFO closure failed to meet primary and secondary end points.[7] Recently, three additional randomized, controlled trials have closed prematurely because of low enrollment.[8] This article reviews the evidence linking migraine and PFO, discusses the results of retrospective and randomized trials, and outlines future research directions. Finally, evidence-based strategies for health care providers managing patients who have migraine and PFO are presented.

MIGRAINEURS: A VULNERABLE POPULATION

Migraine is a genetically based, debilitating neurovascular disorder characterized by prolonged and recurring attacks of severe headache pain[9] that may be accompanied by neurologic and gastrointestinal symptoms. An estimated 28 million Americans experience recurrent migraine headaches;[10] specifically, 17.6% of women and 5.7% of men experience at least one migraine per year.[11] In 30% to 40% of migraineurs, pain is preceded by aura, characterized by transient focal neurologic deficits that usually involve the visual field.[12] Migraine-related symptoms are more common in migraineurs with aura (MA+) than in migraineurs without aura (MA−) (nausea: 67% vs 17%, respectively, $P<.001$; photophobia: 60% vs 33%, respectively, $P = .04$).[13] The diagnostic criteria given in the second edition of the International Classification of Headache Disorders, released by the International Headache Society,[14] are summarized in **Box 1**.

Psychosocial Impacts of Migraine

Migraine headache typically affects persons during their most productive years (25–55 years of age).[15] In one population-based survey, peak migraine prevalence

Department of Cardiovascular Scientific Development, Swedish Medical Center, 500 17th Avenue NE, Suite 303, Seattle, WA 98122, USA; and the University of Washington School of Nursing, 1959 NE, Pacific Street, Seattle, WA 98195, USA
* Corresponding author.
E-mail address: Jill.jesurum@swedish.org (J. Jesurum).

Crit Care Nurs Clin N Am 21 (2009) 471–491
doi:10.1016/j.ccell.2009.07.011
0899-5885/09/$ – see front matter © 2009 Elsevier Inc. All rights reserved.

Box 1
Summary of the International Classification of Headache Disorders diagnostic criteria for migraine headaches

I. Migraine without aura

    A. At least five attacks fulfilling criteria B–D

    B. Headache attacks lasting 4–72 hours (untreated or unsuccessfully treated)

    C. Headaches have at least two of the following characteristics:

        1. Unilateral location

        2. Pulsating quality

        3. Moderate or severe intensity

        4. Aggravation by or causing avoidance of routine physical activity (eg, walking or climbing stairs)

    D. During the headache at least one of the following occurs:

        1. Nausea and/or vomiting

        2. Photophobia and phonophobia

    E. Not attributed to another disorder

II. Migraine with aura

    A. At least two attacks fulfilling criteria B–D

    B. Aura consisting of at least one of the following, but no motor weakness:

        1. Fully reversible visual symptoms including positive features (eg, flickering lights, spots, or lines) and/or negative features (ie, loss of vision)

        2. Fully reversible sensory symptoms including positive features (ie, pins and needles) and/or negative features (ie, numbness)

        3. Fully reversible dysphasic speech disturbance

    C. At least two of the following:

        1. Homonymous visual symptoms and/or unilateral sensory symptoms

        2. At least one aura symptom develops gradually over ≥5 minutes and/or different aura symptoms occur in succession over ≥5 minutes

        3. Each symptom lasts ≥5 and ≤60 minutes

    D. Headache fulfilling criteria B–D for migraine without aura begins during the aura or follows aura within 60 minutes

    E. Not attributed to another disorder

From The International Classification of Headache Disorders: 2nd edition. *Cephalalgia* 2004;24 (Suppl 1):24–6; with permission.

was between the ages of 30 and 39 years and declined thereafter.[16] Migraine has significant negative impacts on productivity.[17] The direct and indirect costs of migraine to the United States economy are estimated at $23 billion per year.[18,19] Migraineurs often develop coping strategies (eg, napping) to remain on the job during a migraine attack,[20] despite being less productive.[21] In addition, during interictal periods migraineurs are less physically active[22] and are more tired than non-migraineurs.[23,24] Major depression and anxiety are common in migraineurs (odds ratios [OR] vs non-migraineurs, 4.5 [95% confidence interval (CI), 3.0–6.9] and

3.2 [95% CI, 2.2–4.6], respectively)[25] and are related to the degree of migraine-related disability.[26,27]

The physical and psychological effects of migraine adversely impact quality of life for patients and their families.[28–30] Migraineurs, especially those with more severe disability, score lower than non-migraineurs on health-related quality-of-life surveys.[30,31] Tietjen and colleagues[27] identified three distinct comorbid constellations of migraine. The migraineur group that was characterized by comorbid depression, anxiety, and fibromyalgia had more disability and lower quality of life than the migraineur group with comorbid hypertension, hyperlipidemia, diabetes, and hypothyroidism or the migraineur group without defining comorbidities.[27] Suicide attempts are more common among persons who suffer migraine than among non-migraineurs (OR 3.0, 95% CI 1.2–8.0),[25] and the presence of aura increases the risk of suicide attempts (relative risk [RR] vs non-migraineurs 5.4, 95% CI 3.1–9.4).[32] Migraine prevention regimens are associated with reduced headache frequency, reduced headache-related disability, and improved quality of life.[33,34] Restoring normal function, in addition to pain relief, now is recognized by the American Academy of Neurology as a primary treatment goal.[35,36]

Neurologic and Cardiovascular Sequelae of Migraine

Migraineurs are at higher risk for ischemic stroke than non-migraineurs (level of evidence A). Migraineurs in the Physicians' Health Study had a relative risk for stroke of 2.0 (95% CI 1.1–3.6).[37] A history of migraine is a significant risk factor for ischemic stroke in women younger than age 35 years.[38] The risk for ischemic stroke is present for migraineurs with and without aura.[39] In the Atherosclerosis Risk in Communities Study,[40] the OR for stroke symptoms for MA+ subjects was 5.46 (95% CI 3.64–8.18); for MA– subjects, the OR for stroke symptoms was 2.45 (95% CI 1.66–3.60).

Migraineurs have an increased risk of infarctions and subclinical lesions in posterior areas of the brain supplied by the basilar artery.[41,42] In contrast, non-migraineurs are more likely to exhibit ischemic stroke in the anterior circulation, particularly in territories supplied by the deep middle cerebral artery (MCA).[43] White matter lesions (WML) are present in migraineurs to a greater extent than in non-migraineurs[44] and are more prevalent in MA+ patients and in migraineurs who have a greater headache frequency.[45] The OR for WML for MA+ patients is 13.7 (95% CI 1.7–112).[41] The risk of WML is increased for younger migraineurs who have no co-existing risk factors for cerebrovascular disease.[46] These WML may be asymptomatic but are associated with reduced cognitive function in the elderly.[47] Migraineurs have been shown to have deficits in reaction time, memory, attention, and mild executive dysfunction during interictal periods compared with age- and gender-matched non-migraineurs, and these deficits are associated with severity, duration, and frequency of migraine attacks.[48–50] Calandre and colleagues[49] found areas of brain hypoperfusion and ischemia in 43% of migraineurs, and the presence of these areas was associated with poorer performance on visual and verbal memory tests relative to non-migraineurs.

Migraineurs may be at greater risk for cardiovascular disease than non-migraineurs. In the Women's Health Study, subjects who had self-reported migraine with aura had hazard ratios of 2.08 (95% CI 1.30–3.31; P = .002) for myocardial infarction, 1.74 (95% CI 1.23–2.46; P = .002) for coronary revascularization, and 1.71 (95% CI 1.16–2.53; P = .007) for angina.[51] In a subsequent analysis, an increased risk of myocardial infarction was related directly to Framingham risk score for MA+ patients; however, there was no increased risk for cardiovascular disease or stroke for MA– patients.[52]

Migraineurs often have additional conditions that may increase their risk for ischemic stroke, and the presence of these conditions can confound a definitive association between migraine and stroke (**Table 1**). Obesity is associated with the prevalence and severity of "transformed migraine," defined as 15 or more headache days per month.[53] The frequency and severity of headaches in episodic and probable migraineurs also are associated with obesity.[54] MacClellan and colleagues[55] reported a sevenfold increase in stroke risk (95% CI 1.3–22.8) in women with probable migraine with visual aura who smoked and used oral contraceptives compared with those who did not smoke or use oral contraceptive. The association between blood pressure and migraine is more controversial. In one study, persons who had high blood pressure were less likely to experience migraine than those who had normal blood pressure (risk ratio 0.56, 95% CI 0.41–0.77)[56]; however, a population-based study showed that a 1-SD increase in diastolic pressure increased migraine risk by 14% in men ($P = .011$) and 30% in women ($P<.0001$).[57] Although migraineurs in the Women's Health Study were less likely to carry the methylene tetrahydrofolate reductase homozygous 677C>T genotype, MA+ subjects with this genotype had a significantly increased risk of ischemic stroke relative to other genotypes (RR 4.2, 95% CI 1.4–12.7, $P = .01$).[58]

Proposed Migraine Pathophysiologic Mechanisms

Cortical spreading depression

The predominant proposed mechanism of migrainous aura is cortical spreading depression (CSD), a wave of neuronal and glial depolarization originating in the visual cortex that results in hyperemia followed by vasoconstriction.[59] Functional MRI in migraineurs during aura showed a focal increase in signal intensity in the occipital cortex, which progressed retinotopically and then diminished.[60] CSD is associated with expression of genes associated with stress, inflammation, and ion transport;[61,62] in addition, CSD can result in disruption of the blood–brain barrier by a matrix metalloproteinase-9–dependent mechanism.[63] In animal models, CSD triggered trigeminal nerve activity consistent with the development of headache pain.[64] Migraineurs also were found to have hyperexcitability of the visual cortex compared with non-migraineur controls.[65,66]

Platelets and migraine

Increased platelet activation and aggregation is an emerging theory to explain CSD and the increased risk of stroke in migraineurs.[67] Both MA+ women (RR 2.88, 95% CI 1.61–3.19)[39] and women who have probable migraine with aura (OR 1.5, 95% CI 1.1–2.0)[55] have an increased risk of ischemic stroke. Increased platelet activation is

Table 1
Comorbid conditions in migraineurs that may increase risk of ischemic stroke (all levels of evidence: B)

Condition	Type of Migraine
Obesity	Presence and severity of transformed migraine[a,53]
	Frequency and severity of episodic migraine[54]
Combined oral contraceptive and tobacco use	Probable MA+[55]
Hypertension	Migraine (no distinction between MA+ and MA−)[57]
Increased platelet activation and aggregation	Migraine (no distinction between MA+ and MA−)[68,70]
Prothrombotic state	Migraine (no distinction between MA+ and MA−)[75,77–79]
Endothelial dysfunction	Migraine (no distinction between MA+ and MA−)[80,81]

Abbreviations: MA+, migraine with aura; MA−, migraine without aura.
[a] Defined as 15 or more headache days per month.

theorized to trigger headache symptoms through the release of inflammatory and pro-aggregatory mediators and may produce transient ischemia caused by microaggregates impairing the cerebral microcirculation.[68,69] Migraineurs showed increased peripheral blood cell expression of the platelet-related genes cyclooxygenase-2, glycoprotein IIb, and c-fos during an acute attack, relative to non-migraineurs and individuals with other neurologic diseases (epilepsy, bipolar disorder).[67] Internal jugular vein levels of platelet-activating factor were increased in MA− subjects ($n = 5$) early in headache when compared with the end of the headache period.[70] During interictal periods, migraineurs have increased circulating P-selectin (a biomarker of platelet activation) and platelet-leukocyte aggregates compared with non-migraineurs.[68] Platelet surface P-selectin expression is increased in MA− patients relative to controls ($P = .001$), and there is a trend toward an increase in MA+ patients relative to controls ($P = .08$).[71] CD40 ligand (CD40L) is a transmembrane protein related to tumor necrosis factor alpha. Both CD40L and its receptor, CD40, are expressed on endothelial cells, smooth muscle cells, monocytes, macrophages, and platelets. Platelets are a primary origin for circulating CD40L, which is translocated rapidly to the platelet surface following platelet activation and subsequently is cleaved from the platelet.[72] Binding of CD40L to CD40 on platelets can result in release of reactive oxygen and nitrogen species[73] and increased platelet aggregation.[74]

Measures of blood coagulation also are increased in migraineurs. Migraineurs had shorter platelet hemostasis time and collagen-induced thrombus formation time than did age- and sex-matched non-migraineurs, indicative of increased platelet aggregation.[75] Von Willebrand factor levels and activity also were higher in migraineurs than in non-migraineurs,[75] consistent with an earlier investigation.[76] Prothrombin factor 1.2 was higher in MA+ patients than in MA− patients and non-migraineurs.[77] Migraineurs with aura had a 6.1% (3/49) prevalence of factor V Leiden, but this prevalence did not differ from that in MA− patients (1/57, 1.7%) or non-migraineurs (3/106, 2.8%).[78] More recently, migraineurs were reported to be more likely than non-migraineurs to have a history of venous thromboembolism (18.9% vs 7.6%, respectively; $P = .031$ when adjusted for age and sex).[79]

Endothelial dysfunction, which affects both platelet activity and thrombosis, also may play a role in the increased stroke risk for migraineurs.[80,81] Flow-mediated dilation was significantly reduced in migraineurs compared with non-migraineurs.[80] The homozygous Glu298Asp genotype of endothelial nitric oxide synthase was three times more common in MA+ patients than in MA− patients and was twice as common as in non-migraineurs.[82] Circulating endothelial precursor cell number and function were reduced in migraineurs relative to non-migraineurs,[81] perhaps increasing the risk of cardiovascular disease. Taken together, a pro-platelet aggregation and prothrombotic state exists in migraineurs that may predispose them to ischemic stroke.

PATENT FORAMEN OVALE

The foramen ovale is an opening in the interatrial septum resulting from incomplete coverage of the ostium secundum—an opening within the septum primum—by the septum secundum. **Fig. 1** shows a PFO. The foramen ovale serves as a one-way valve for physiologic right-to-left shunting (RLS) of oxygenated blood in utero. Blood from the placenta enters the right atrium through the inferior vena cava and crosses the foramen ovale into the systemic circulation. Postnatal lung expansion and initiation of the pulmonary circulation reverses the atrial pressure gradient, causing functional closure of the foramen ovale. Fibrosis follows closure, and complete fusion of the interatrial septae occurs by 2 years of age in most individuals.[83] If the septae fail to fuse,

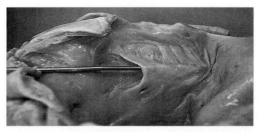

Fig. 1. Autopsy specimen of patent foramen ovale, as seen from the left atrium. (*From* Desai AJ, Fuller CJ, Jesurum JT, Reisman M. Patent foramen ovale and cerebrovascular diseases. Nat Clin Pract Cardiovasc Med 2006:3(8):447–55; with permission).

the resulting PFO is a potential tunnel that can be opened by reversal of the interatrial pressure gradient or by an intracardiac catheter.

Familial PFO prevalence is consistent with autosomal dominant inheritance.[84] Female siblings of stroke patients with PFO are more likely to have PFO than siblings of stroke patients without PFO (OR 9.8, $P<.01$).[85] Interestingly, this finding was not seen in male siblings of stroke patients with PFO. Autopsy studies showed the presence of PFO in 17% to 29% of the general population.[86–88] Noninvasive population-based studies showed a similar prevalence of PFO in the general population, ranging from 17%[89] to 26%.[84] No sex difference was seen in either study. The prevalence of PFO declined with age, from 30% among persons younger than 30 years to 20% among persons older than 80 years; however, PFO diameter increased with age.[88]

Detection of Patent Foramen Ovale

The current reference standard for detection of PFO is contrast-enhanced transesophageal echocardiography (c-TEE), which allows quantitative assessment of the degree of intracardiac shunting and visualization of the cardiac anatomy.[90] The sensitivity of c-TEE in detecting a PFO may be increased most effectively by a Valsalva maneuver (VM); however, patients may be unable to perform an adequate VM because of the sedation required. Transthoracic echocardiography (TTE) also is used in PFO detection, but its sensitivity and specificity are compromised by inadequate visualization of cardiac structures.[91] Transcranial Doppler (TCD) is comparable to c-TEE for detecting PFO-related RLS.[92] Unlike TEE, TCD does not require sedation of the patient, thus ensuring better performance of VM. Power motion-mode TCD produced sensitivity and specificity comparable to that of TEE in diagnosis of PFO when compared with the ability to pass a guide wire across the atrial septum in the catheterization laboratory (TCD: sensitivity 98%, specificity 33%; TEE: sensitivity 91%, specificity 33%).[93] TCD does not provide any information concerning interatrial septum morphology or PFO diameter, however. Detection of RLS with c-TCD alone does not confirm the diagnosis of PFO, because RLS of another cardiac or extracardiac source may be present. This limitation can be overcome with concurrent TTE to confirm a cardiac source of RLS.[94] Although bilateral MCA detection of PFO by TCD is optimal, unilateral MCA monitoring is equivalent in detecting large RLS following performance of a VM.[95] Vertebrobasilar detection of medium or large RLS by TCD showed 84% sensitivity and 100% specificity relative to right MCA detection.[96]

Patent Foramen Ovale and Cryptogenic Stroke

More than 40% of ischemic strokes that occur in people younger than age 55 years are cryptogenic, in which no risk factors (eg, hypertension or atrial fibrillation) are present.[97] PFO is more prevalent in patients who have cryptogenic stroke than in those who have stroke of known etiology (61% vs 19%).[98] A PFO may serve as a conduit for paradoxical cerebral embolism that could be the causal mechanism for some cryptogenic strokes. A 13% to 56% prevalence of PFO has been reported among young patients who have suffered ischemic stroke.[99–104] The risk of stroke in persons younger than age 55 years with a PFO was greater than in age-matched controls without a PFO (OR 3.10, 95% CI 2.29–4.21).[105] A recent study showed an association of PFO with cryptogenic stroke among older patients (aged >55 years) (OR 2.92, 95% CI 1.70–5.01, $P<.001$).[106] The risk of stroke recurrence within 3 years among patients who had PFO was 7.2% and increased to 16.3% among patients who had cryptogenic stroke.[107] Risk of stroke also is increased with large PFO diameter (>2 mm)[108,109] and large magnitude of RLS measured by TEE or TCD.[107,110,111]

PFO may be associated with other risk factors for stroke. Atrial septal aneurysm (ASA) is defined as a hypermobile septum primum with an excursion of 10 mm or greater into either atrium.[112] Although the prevalence of isolated ASA is less than 1% in the general population,[112] the prevalence in patients who have suffered cryptogenic stroke is 4% to 25%.[99] The coexistence of ASA with PFO increases the OR for stroke to 15.59 (95% CI 2.83–85.87).[105] The presence of both PFO and ASA is a significant predictor for recurrent stroke (hazard ratio 4.17, 95% CI 1.47–11.84).[107,113] Inherited prothrombotic disorders, particularly the prothrombin gene G20210 mutation, have been associated with PFO in patients who have suffered cryptogenic stroke.[114–116] In one study, patients who had suffered cryptogenic stroke and who had a large PFO were more likely to have circulating antiphospholipid antibodies than those who did not have a PFO.[117]

The source of paradoxical cerebral emboli in patients who have PFO is unknown; however, Cramer and colleagues[98] reported that the incidence of pelvic deep vein thrombosis was higher in patients who had cryptogenic stroke (20%) and in patients who had cryptogenic stroke and PFO (22%) than in patients who had stroke of determined origin (4%; $P<.025$). Patients who had cryptogenic stroke were significantly younger and had fewer risk factors for atherosclerosis than those who had stroke of known cause. The prevalence of PFO was 61% in the cryptogenic stroke group and 19% in those who had a stroke of determined origin. The finding that most patients who had cryptogenic stroke and pelvic deep vein thrombosis also had a PFO supports paradoxical embolism as the stroke mechanism.

PATENT FORAMEN OVALE AND MIGRAINE: A CAUSAL LINK

Some investigators have recognized an association between migraine headache and PFO.[1] The prevalence of PFO is estimated as 47% to 67% in MA+ patients, as 23% to 47% in MA– patients, and as 17% to 25% among controls.[3–5,118] The odds ratio of having migraine in the presence of PFO with moderate or large RLS was 7.78 (95% CI 2.53–29.3, $P<.001$).[4] The presence of PFO and migraine with aura may be genetically linked.[119,120] It has been speculated that interatrial transit of microemboli or vasoactive compounds through the PFO can lead to migrainous symptoms, ischemic stroke, or both.[4] Nearly half of MA+ patients in one survey reported VM-provoking activities as triggers for migraine attacks,[121] and they were more likely to have a large amount of embolic conductance, suggestive of large RLS, as measured by TCD. Interestingly, VM-provoking activities (eg, exercise, sexual activity, coughing) were reported as migraine triggers by 15% of migraineurs who were not screened for RLS.[122]

The association between migraine and PFO is not universally accepted. Gori and colleagues[123] reported that the extent of RLS did not correlate with the severity of migraine with aura. Rundek and colleagues[124] found no difference in the prevalence of PFO between migraineurs and non-migraineurs in the Northern Manhattan Study cohort (14.6% vs 15.0%, respectively, $P = .9$); in addition, only 2% of subjects had both PFO and migraine. It should be noted that the mean age in the Northern Manhattan Study sample was 69 ($\pm$10) years, outside the period of peak migraine prevalence,[15] and PFO was diagnosed by TTE.

EFFECT OF PATENT FORAMEN OVALE CLOSURE ON MIGRAINE FREQUENCY AND SYMPTOMS

Options for preventing recurrent cryptogenic stroke secondary to PFO are limited. Antiplatelet (ie, aspirin) or anticoagulant (ie, warfarin) therapy is the current standard of care (level of evidence B).[125] There is no evidence to show that antiplatelet therapy is superior to anticoagulant therapy in secondary stroke prevention for persons who have PFO (hazard ratio 1.3, 95% CI 0.6–2.6).[109] Transcatheter closure of PFO using an implantable device to occlude the PFO to prevent recurrent stroke was covered by a Humanitarian Device Exemption (HDE); however, the US Food and Drug Administration (FDA) withdrew the HDE in 2006 when it became apparent that more than 4000 patients (the maximum number for an HDE designation) conceivably could use the closure procedure each year.[126]

The majority of early transcatheter PFO closures were performed to prevent recurrent stroke or decompression illness in divers; migraine relief was a coincidental finding.[1,127] In several retrospective, nonrandomized studies, transcatheter closure of PFO resulted in complete resolution or marked reduction in migraine frequency (level of evidence B) (**Table 2**).[6,127–130] Reisman and colleagues[6] reported complete migraine resolution in 56% of patients, and 14% of patients reported a significant (>50%) reduction in migraine frequency. In the same study, patients reported an 80% reduction in the mean number of migraine episodes per month after PFO closure (6.8 $\pm$ 9.6 before closure vs 1.4 $\pm$ 3.4 after closure, $P<.001$). In a subsequent analysis from this research group,[94] the presence of residual RLS following PFO closure was not associated with lack of migraine relief ($\leq$50% reduction in migraine days per month). The authors hypothesized that PFO closure reduced the degree of RLS below a "neuronal threshold" that may have resulted in migraine relief. In addition, MA+ patients who underwent PFO closure were 4.5 times more likely to experience migraine relief than MA– patients.[94]

The results of retrospective studies showing migraine relief following transcatheter PFO closure resulted in the design of several prospective device trials. Trials listed on clinicaltrials.gov,[8] as well as other trials, are shown in **Table 3**. Migraine Intervention with STARFlex Technology (MIST) is the only randomized, double-blind trial of PFO closure and migraine treatment completed and published to date.[7] The MIST trial failed to meet the primary end point of complete migraine resolution 6 months after procedure; 3 of 74 implanted patients and 3 of 73 sham-procedure patients experienced complete relief ($P = .51$). The secondary end point of headache days per 3 months also did not differ between the two groups, either in the intent-to-treat or the per-protocol populations ($P = .79$ and $P = .85$, respectively). Only when two outliers were eliminated from the analysis was a 37% reduction in headache days per 3 months seen in the implant group, compared with 26% in the sham-procedure group ($P = .027$).[7] Other prospective trials of transcatheter PFO closure in migraine have been discontinued because of insufficient enrollment.[8,131,132] In a very small randomized, open-label trial, Sarens and colleagues[132] reported a significant decrease in MA+ days per month at 6 months following device implantation ($n = 4$; 4.8 $\pm$ 3.4 vs 2.3 $\pm$ 3.3 days, $P = .011$), whereas patients receiving 160 mg aspirin per day for 6 months had a comparable decrease in MA+ days per month that was not significant ($n = 5$; 4.2 $\pm$ 3.6 vs 1.9 $\pm$ 2.9 days,

Table 2
Major publications of transcatheter PFO closure for migraine prevention[a]

Authors	Number (% Female)	Mean Age in Years (SD)	Number with MA+ (%)	Mean Follow-up	Migraines Resolved (%)	Reduced Severity or Frequency (%)	Unchanged (%)
Wilmshurst et al (2000)[127]	21 (48)	NA	16 (76)	1.5–32 months (range)	48 (44 MA+; 60 MA−)	38 (50 MA+; 0 MA−)	14 (6 MA+; 40 MA−)
Schwerzmann et al (2004)[128]	48 (65)	MA+ 49 (11); MA− 42 (12)	37 (77)	1.7 year	NA	54 MA+; 62 MA−	3 MA+ and large residual shunt
Azarbal et al (2005)[153]	37 (66)	NA	20 (54)	12 months	75 MA+; 40 MA−	5 MA+; 40 MA−	NA
Reisman et al (2005)[6]	57 (67)	47 (12)	39 (68)	37 weeks	56 (54 MA+; 62 MA−)	14 (14 MA+; 15 MA−)	30 (32 MA+; 23 MA−)
Anzola et al (2006)[130]	50 (82)	NA	40 (80)	12 months	36	52	8
Slavin et al (2007)[129]	50 (75)	46 (12)	40 (80)	30 months	64 (68 MA+; 50 MA−)	21 (13 MA+; 40 MA−)	NA
Dubiel et al (2008)[154]	46 (76)	44 (14)	24 (52)	38 months	24 (33 MA+; 14 MA−)	63 (58 MA+; 68 MA−)	NA

[a] Most of these studies were neither prospective nor randomized.

Table 3
Prospective trials of PFO closure in migraine (as of February 2009)

Trial	Sponsor	Location(s)	Design	Status
MIST: Migraine Intervention with STARFlex Technology	NMT Medical	United Kingdom	Randomized, double-blind	Completed[7]
MIST II PFO: Migraine Trial with BioSTAR Bioabsorbable Septal Repair Implant	NMT Medical	United States	Randomized, double-blind	Active; not recruiting (low enrollment)
STOP PAIN: Septal Closure of PFO—Does it Prevent Migraine?	St. Jude Medical	Germany	Randomized, double-blind	Suspended (low enrollment, ethical concerns)
ESCAPE Migraine Trial	St. Jude Medical	United States	Randomized, double-blind	Active; not recruiting (low enrollment)[131]
FORMAT: Patent Foramen Ovale Closure to Reduce Migraine Attacks	CARDIA	Belgium	Randomized, open-labeled	Suspended (low enrollment, device discontinued)
The Paradigm II Trial: PFX closure system in subjects with cryptogenic stroke, transient ischemic attack, migraine or decompression illness	Cierra	Germany	Nonrandomized	Completed
PFx closure system in subjects with cryptogenic stroke, transient ischemic attack, migraine or Decompression illness	Cierra	Germany, Belgium, France	Nonrandomized	Suspended
PREMIUM: Prospective Randomized Investigation to Evaluate Incidence of Headache Reduction in Subjects with Migraine and PFO Using the AMPLATZER PFO Occluder Compared with Medical Management	AGA Medical	United States	Randomized, double-blind	Active; recruiting subjects
PRIMA: PFO Repair In Migraine with Aura	AGA Medical	Canada, Switzerland, Germany, UK	Randomized, double-blind	Active; recruiting subjects

Abbreviations: MA+, migraine with aura; MA−, migraine without aura; NA, data not available.
Compiled from: clinicaltrials.gov, literature, and device manufacturer Web sites.

$P = .16$). At this time, the FDA has not approved transcatheter PFO closure for migraine relief outside of ongoing randomized trials.

Some patients may experience new-onset or increased frequency of migraines following PFO closure.[133,134] One potential cause for new or increased migraines is nickel hypersensitivity, because the nitinol alloy used in closure devices is 55% nickel.[135] Blood nickel levels have been found to increase significantly following PFO device implantation and to decrease to baseline following endothelialization of the device at 12 months.[136] Pericarditis and other cardiac adverse events have been reported in nickel-sensitive patients following PFO closure;[134,135] therefore, nickel hypersensitivity should be a contraindication to PFO closure (level of evidence B).

FUTURE DIRECTIONS

More research is needed to define the mechanisms of migraine in persons who have RLS. There have been few comparisons of atrial septal anatomy between migraineurs and non-migraineurs who have PFO. In patients undergoing transcatheter PFO closure, migraineurs were more likely to have large RLS at rest and following calibrated respiratory strain than non-migraineurs, despite similar PFO diameter and tunnel length measured by intracardiac echocardiography.[137] A recent study using intracardiac echocardiography and transcranial Doppler also found a secondary source of RLS in 20% of patients undergoing PFO closure.[138] At late follow-up, 93% of patients who had secondary RLS and 44% of patients who did not have secondary RLS had residual RLS ($P = .002$). The presence of secondary RLS could explain in part why 7% of the subjects randomly assigned to PFO closure in the MIST trial had no detectable PFO in the catheterization laboratory.[7]

More research is needed to identify comorbid factors that can predispose migraineurs who have PFO and those who do not have PFO to stroke or signal-silent brain lesions. The prevalence of PFO may be as high as 25% in the general population,[88] and many of these individuals may not have stroke or migraine;[124,139] therefore, other factors may play additive or synergistic roles. Vasomotor reactivity to hyper- and hypocapnia is altered in migraineurs,[140] and this alteration could facilitate the transit of microemboli in persons who have hypercoagulable states or increased platelet aggregation to the posterior circulation. As many as 69% of persons who have obstructive sleep apnea have PFO;[141] in addition, migraineurs are more likely than non-migraineurs to report excessive daytime sleepiness.[23,24] The prevalence of obstructive sleep apnea in migraineurs is unknown. Finally, altered cognitive function in migraineurs may be indicative of WML. The contribution of PFO to cognitive dysfunction in migraineurs is currently unknown.

APPLICATIONS TO CLINICAL PRACTICE

Counseling patients who have migraine and PFO presents a clinical dilemma. Randomized trials are essential for determining the efficacy of transcatheter PFO closure in reducing migraine frequency; however, many patients are reluctant to volunteer lest they be randomly assigned to placebo. It should be noted that a placebo effect of up to 40% is present in migraine rescue or prophylactic medication trials,[142,143] and the patients undergoing the sham procedure in MIST experienced a 26% reduction in migraine days.[7] In addition, the inclusion/exclusion criteria for randomized trials may hamper enrollment because of stringency or excessive participant burden (eg, maintenance of online headache diaries for 90 days).

Table 4 lists evidence-based strategies for patients who have PFO and migraine headaches. Prevention of stroke is of primary concern, because migraineurs who

Table 4
Evidence-based guidelines for stroke prevention and migraine prevention/treatment for patients who have migraine and PFO

Purpose	Guideline	Level of Evidence
Stroke Prevention	Risk factor modification[145] • Weight • Blood pressure • Glycemic control • Hyperlipidemia control	A
	Anticoagulant or aspirin therapy[109,146]	A
	Check post-treatment platelet reactivity to aspirin, particularly in women[147,148]	B
Migraine Prevention and Treatment	Trigger control[121,122]	A
	Use of preventive and rescue medications as tolerated	A
	Topiramate[150]	A
	Beta-blockers[149]	A
	Sodium valproate[155]	A
	Triptans[151]	A
	Nonsteroidal anti-inflammatory drugs ± triptans[152,156]	B

have large RLS at rest are at higher risk for recurrent stroke.[144] Aggressive risk factor management (smoking cessation and weight, blood pressure, and glycemic control) should be undertaken (level of evidence A).[145] Treatment with aspirin (325 mg) or warfarin (to attain an International Normalized Ratio between 1.4 and 2.8) had equal efficacy in reducing the risk of recurrent stroke in persons who had PFO (level of evidence A).[109] There is no evidence to date that clopidogrel confers any advantage over aspirin or warfarin for stroke prevention in this cohort. Aspirin, 100 mg on alternate days, has been shown to reduce the risk of stroke in women (RR 0.83, 95% CI 0.69–0.99, $P = .04$) without affecting the risk of myocardial infarction (RR 1.02, 95% CI, 0.84–1.25, $P = .83$).[146] Women may be more likely to have high aspirin platelet reactivity after treatment;[147,148] therefore, testing for platelet reactivity during aspirin treatment may be advisable.

Patients should recognize their unique migraine triggers (eg, sleep deprivation, fasting) and avoid them.[121,122] If tolerated, preventive medications such as topiramate or beta-blockers can be prescribed.[149,150] Patients may need to try different triptans or combinations with other medications (eg, naproxen sodium) before they find the most effective one for their migraines.[151,152] It should be emphasized to patients that randomized trials are the only way to advance the science of migraine treatment by PFO closure; therefore, health care professionals must encourage patients' participation.

SUMMARY

Prospective evidence to recommend transcatheter PFO closure as a migraine treatment is lacking. It is incumbent on health care providers to assist their patients in understanding the results of research studies and to encourage them to participate in well-designed randomized clinical trials.

REFERENCES

1. Wilmshurst P, Nightingale S. Relationship between migraine and cardiac and pulmonary right-to-left shunts. Clin Sci (Lond) 2001;100(2):215–20.

2. Dalla Volta G, Guindani M, Zavarise P, et al. Prevalence of patent foramen ovale in a large series of patients with migraine with aura, migraine without aura and cluster headache, and relationship with clinical phenotype. J Headache Pain 2005;6(4):328–30.

3. Domitrz I, Mieszkowski J, Kwiecinski H. [The prevalence of patent foramen ovale in patients with migraine]. Neurol Neurochir Pol 2004;38(2):89–92 [in Polish].

4. Schwerzmann M, Nedeltchev K, Lagger F, et al. Prevalence and size of directly detected patent foramen ovale in migraine with aura. Neurology 2005;65:1415–8.

5. Anzola GP, Magoni M, Guindani M, et al. Potential source of cerebral embolism in migraine with aura: a transcranial Doppler study. Neurology 1999;52(8):1622–5.

6. Reisman M, Christofferson RD, Jesurum J, et al. Migraine headache relief after transcatheter closure of patent foramen ovale. J Am Coll Cardiol 2005;45(4):493–5.

7. Dowson A, Mullen MJ, Peatfield R, et al. Migraine intervention with STARFlex technology (MIST) trial: a prospective, multicenter, double-blind, sham-controlled trial to evaluate the effectiveness of patent foramen ovale closure with STARFlex septal repair implant to resolve refractory migraine headache. Circulation 2008;117(11):1397–404.

8. National Library of Medicine. Available at: clinicaltrials.gov. Accessed October 22, 2008.

9. Kwong WJ, Pathak DS. Validation of the eleven-point pain scale in the measurement of migraine headache pain. Cephalalgia 2007;27(4):336–42.

10. Lipton RB, Stewart WF, Diamond S, et al. Prevalence and burden of migraine in the United States: data from the American Migraine Study II. Headache 2001;41(7):646–57.

11. Cook NR, Bensenor IM, Lotufo PA, et al. Migraine and coronary heart disease in women and men. Headache 2002;42(8):715–27.

12. Cutrer FM, Huerter K. Migraine aura. Neurologist 2007;13(3):118–25.

13. Quintela E, Castillo J, Munoz P, et al. Premonitory and resolution symptoms in migraine: a prospective study in 100 unselected patients. Cephalalgia 2006;26(9):1051–60.

14. Headache classification subcommittee, International Headache Society. The international classification of headache disorders: 2nd edition. Cephalalgia 2004;24(Suppl 1):9–160.

15. Leonardi M, Steiner TJ, Scher AT, et al. The global burden of migraine: measuring disability in headache disorders with WHO's Classification of Functioning, Disability and Health (ICF). J Headache Pain 2005;6(6):429–40.

16. Bigal ME, Liberman JN, Lipton RB. Age-dependent prevalence and clinical features of migraine. Neurology 2006;67(2):246–51.

17. Aukerman G, Knutson D, Miser WF. Management of the acute migraine headache. Am Fam Physician 2002;66(11):2123–30.

18. Hawkins K, Wang S, Rupnow MF. Indirect cost burden of migraine in the United States. J Occup Environ Med 2007;49(4):368–74.

19. Hawkins K, Wang S, Rupnow M. Direct cost burden among insured US employees with migraine. Headache 2008;48(4):553–63.

20. Berry PA. Migraine disorder: workplace implications and solutions. AAOHN J 2007;55(2):51–6.

21. Moloney MF, Strickland OL, DeRossett SE, et al. The experiences of midlife women with migraines. J Nurs Scholarsh 2006;38(3):278–85.

22. Bigal ME, Bigal JM, Betti M, et al. Evaluation of the impact of migraine and episodic tension-type headache on the quality of life and performance of a university student population. Headache 2001;41(7):710–9.

23. Stronks DL, Tulen JH, Bussmann JB, et al. Interictal daily functioning in migraine. Cephalalgia 2004;24(4):271–9.

24. Barbanti P, Fabbrini G, Aurilia C, et al. A case-control study on excessive daytime sleepiness in episodic migraine. Cephalalgia 2007;27(10):1115–9.

25. Breslau N, Davis GC. Migraine, physical health and psychiatric disorder: a prospective epidemiologic study in young adults. J Psychiatr Res 1993;27(2): 211–21.

26. Jelinski SE, Magnusson JE, Becker WJ. Factors associated with depression in patients referred to headache specialists. Neurology 2007;68(7):489–95.

27. Tietjen GE, Herial NA, Hardgrove J, et al. Migraine comorbidity constellations. Headache 2007;47(6):857–65.

28. Lipton RB, Stewart WF, Sawyer J, et al. Clinical utility of an instrument assessing migraine disability: the migraine disability assessment (MIDAS) questionnaire. Headache 2001;41(9):854–61.

29. Meletiche DM, Lofland JH, Young WB. Quality-of-life differences between patients with episodic and transformed migraine. Headache 2001;41(6):573–8.

30. Lipton RB, Liberman JN, Kolodner KB, et al. Migraine headache disability and health-related quality-of-life: a population-based case-control study from England. Cephalalgia 2003;23(6):441–50.

31. Patel NV, Bigal ME, Kolodner KB, et al. Prevalence and impact of migraine and probable migraine in a health plan. Neurology 2004;63(8):1432–8.

32. Breslau N, Davis GC, Andreski P. Migraine, psychiatric disorders, and suicide attempts: an epidemiologic study of young adults. Psychiatry Res 1991;37(1): 11–23.

33. Bordini CA, Mariano da Silva H, Garbelini RP, et al. Effect of preventive treatment on health-related quality of life in episodic migraine. J Headache Pain 2005;6(5): 387–91.

34. D'Amico D, Solari A, Usai S, et al. Improvement in quality of life and activity limitations in migraine patients after prophylaxis. A prospective longitudinal multicentre study. Cephalalgia 2006;26(6):691–6.

35. Silberstein SD, Rosenberg J. Multispecialty consensus on diagnosis and treatment of headache. Neurology 2000;54(8):1553.

36. Wenzel R, Dortch M, Cady R, et al. Migraine headache misconceptions: barriers to effective care. Pharmacotherapy 2004;24(5):638–48.

37. Buring JE, Hebert P, Romero J, et al. Migraine and subsequent risk of stroke in the Physicians' Health Study. Arch Neurol 1995;52(2):129–34.

38. Carolei A, Marini C, De Matteis G. History of migraine and risk of cerebral ischaemia in young adults. The Italian National Research Council Study Group on Stroke in the Young. Lancet 1996;347(9014):1503–6.

39. Etminan M, Takkouche B, Isorna FC, et al. Risk of ischaemic stroke in people with migraine: systematic review and meta-analysis of observational studies. BMJ 2005;330(7482):63–6.

40. Stang PE, Carson AP, Rose KM, et al. Headache, cerebrovascular symptoms, and stroke: the atherosclerosis risk in communities study. Neurology 2005; 64(9):1573–7.

41. Kruit MC, van Buchem MA, Hofman PA, et al. Migraine as a risk factor for subclinical brain lesions. JAMA 2004;291(4):427–34.

42. Kruit MC, Launer LJ, Ferrari MD, et al. Infarcts in the posterior circulation territory in migraine. The population-based MRI CAMERA study. Brain 2005;128(Pt 9): 2068–77.
43. Milhaud D, Bogousslavsky J, van Melle G, et al. Ischemic stroke and active migraine. Neurology 2001;57(10):1805–11.
44. Robbins L, Friedman H. MRI in migraineurs. Headache 1992;32(10):507–8.
45. Gozke E, Ore O, Dortcan N, et al. Cranial magnetic resonance imaging findings in patients with migraine. Headache 2004;44(2):166–9.
46. Swartz RH, Kern RZ. Migraine is associated with magnetic resonance imaging white matter abnormalities: a meta-analysis. Arch Neurol 2004; 61(9):1366–8.
47. Longstreth WT Jr, Manolio TA, Arnold A, et al. Clinical correlates of white matter findings on cranial magnetic resonance imaging of 3301 elderly people. The Cardiovascular Health Study. Stroke 1996;27(8):1274–82.
48. Riva D, Aggio F, Vago C, et al. Cognitive and behavioural effects of migraine in childhood and adolescence. Cephalalgia 2006;26(5):596–603.
49. Calandre EP, Bembibre J, Arnedo ML, et al. Cognitive disturbances and regional cerebral blood flow abnormalities in migraine patients: their relationship with the clinical manifestations of the illness. Cephalalgia 2002;22(4):291–302.
50. Camarda C, Monastero R, Pipia C, et al. Interictal executive dysfunction in migraineurs without aura: relationship with duration and intensity of attacks. Cephalalgia 2007;27(10):1094–100.
51. Kurth T, Gaziano JM, Cook NR, et al. Migraine and risk of cardiovascular disease in women. JAMA 2006;296(3):283–91.
52. Kurth T, Schurks M, Logroscino G, et al. Migraine, vascular risk, and cardiovascular events in women: prospective cohort study. BMJ 2008;337:a636.
53. Bigal ME, Lipton RB. Obesity is a risk factor for transformed migraine but not chronic tension-type headache. Neurology 2006;67(2):252–7.
54. Bigal ME, Tsang A, Loder E, et al. Body mass index and episodic headaches: a population-based study. Arch Intern Med 2007;167(18):1964–70.
55. MacClellan LR, Giles W, Cole J, et al. Probable migraine with visual aura and risk of ischemic stroke: the stroke prevention in young women study. Stroke 2007; 38(9):2438–45.
56. Wiehe M, Fuchs SC, Moreira LB, et al. Migraine is more frequent in individuals with optimal and normal blood pressure: a population-based study. J Hypertens 2002;20(7):1303–6.
57. Gudmundsson LS, Thorgeirsson G, Sigfusson N, et al. Migraine patients have lower systolic but higher diastolic blood pressure compared with controls in a population-based study of 21,537 subjects. The Reykjavik Study. Cephalalgia 2006;26(4):436–44.
58. Schurks M, Zee RY, Buring JE, et al. Interrelationships among the MTHFR 677C>T polymorphism, migraine, and cardiovascular disease. Neurology 2008;71(7):505–13.
59. Sanchez-del-Rio M, Reuter U. Migraine aura: new information on underlying mechanisms. Curr Opin Neurol 2004;17(3):289–93.
60. Hadjikhani N, Sanchez Del Rio M, Wu O, et al. Mechanisms of migraine aura revealed by functional MRI in human visual cortex. Proc Natl Acad Sci U S A 2001; 98(8):4687–92.
61. Choudhuri R, Cui L, Yong C, et al. Cortical spreading depression and gene regulation: relevance to migraine. Ann Neurol 2002;51(4):499–506.

62. Urbach A, Bruehl C, Witte OW. Microarray-based long-term detection of genes differentially expressed after cortical spreading depression. Eur J Neurosci 2006;24(3):841–56.

63. Gursoy-Ozdemir Y, Qiu J, Matsuoka N, et al. Cortical spreading depression activates and upregulates MMP-9. J Clin Invest 2004;113(10):1447–55.

64. Bolay H, Reuter U, Dunn AK, et al. Intrinsic brain activity triggers trigeminal meningeal afferents in a migraine model. Nat Med 2002;8(2):136–42.

65. Battelli L, Black KR, Wray SH. Transcranial magnetic stimulation of visual area V5 in migraine. Neurology 2002;58(7):1066–9.

66. Khedr EM, Ahmed MA, Mohamed KA. Motor and visual cortical excitability in migraineurs patients with or without aura: transcranial magnetic stimulation. Neurophysiol Clin 2006;36(1):13–8.

67. Hershey AD, Tang Y, Powers SW, et al. Genomic abnormalities in patients with migraine and chronic migraine: preliminary blood gene expression suggests platelet abnormalities. Headache 2004;44(10):994–1004.

68. Zeller JA, Frahm K, Baron R, et al. Platelet-leukocyte interaction and platelet activation in migraine: a link to ischemic stroke? J Neurol Neurosurg Psychiatry 2004;75(7):984–7.

69. Fujita S. Effects of correcting platelet hyper-aggregability on prevention of migraine with aura manifested by scintillating scotoma and on migraine outcome using the MIDAS scale. Headache Care 2006;3(2):65–72.

70. Sarchielli P, Alberti A, Coppola F, et al. Platelet-activating factor (PAF) in internal jugular venous blood of migraine without aura patients assessed during migraine attacks. Cephalalgia 2004;24(8):623–30.

71. Zeller JA, Lindner V, Frahm K, et al. Platelet activation and platelet-leucocyte interaction in patients with migraine. Subtype differences and influence of triptans. Cephalalgia 2005;25(7):536–41.

72. Aukrust P, Muller F, Ueland T, et al. Enhanced levels of soluble and membrane-bound CD40 ligand in patients with unstable angina. Possible reflection of T lymphocyte and platelet involvement in the pathogenesis of acute coronary syndromes. Circulation 1999;100(6):614–20.

73. Chakrabarti S, Varghese S, Vitseva O, et al. CD40 ligand influences platelet release of reactive oxygen intermediates. Arterioscler Thromb Vasc Biol 2005;25(11):2428–34.

74. Mason PJ, Chakrabarti S, Albers AA, et al. Plasma, serum, and platelet expression of CD40 ligand in adults with cardiovascular disease. Am J Cardiol 2005;96(10):1365–9.

75. Tietjen GE, Al-Qasmi MM, Athanas K, et al. Altered hemostasis in migraineurs studied with a dynamic flow system. Thromb Res 2007;119(2):217–22.

76. Tietjen GE, Al-Qasmi MM, Athanas K, et al. Increased von Willebrand factor in migraine. Neurology 2001;57(2):334–6.

77. Hering-Hanit R, Friedman Z, Schlesinger I, et al. Evidence for activation of the coagulation system in migraine with aura. Cephalalgia 2001;21(2):137–9.

78. Corral J, Iniesta JA, Gonzalez-Conejero R, et al. Migraine and prothrombotic genetic risk factors. Cephalalgia 1998;18(5):257–60.

79. Schwaiger J, Kiechl S, Stockner H, et al. Burden of atherosclerosis and risk of venous thromboembolism in patients with migraine. Neurology 2008;71(12):937–43.

80. Yetkin E, Ozisik H, Ozcan C, et al. Decreased endothelium-dependent vasodilatation in patients with migraine: a new aspect to vascular pathophysiology of migraine. Coron Artery Dis 2006;17(1):29–33.

81. Lee ST, Chu K, Jung KH, et al. Decreased number and function of endothelial progenitor cells in patients with migraine. Neurology 2008;70(17):1510–7.
82. Borroni B, Rao R, Liberini P, et al. Endothelial nitric oxide synthase (Glu298Asp) polymorphism is an independent risk factor for migraine with aura. Headache 2006;46(10):1575–9.
83. Kerut EK, Norfleet WT, Plotnick GD, et al. Patent foramen ovale: a review of associated conditions and the impact of physiological size. J Am Coll Cardiol 2001; 38(3):613–23.
84. Meissner I, Whisnant JP, Khandheria BK, et al. Prevalence of potential risk factors for stroke assessed by transesophageal echocardiography and carotid ultrasonography: the SPARC study. Stroke prevention: assessment of risk in a community. Mayo Clin Proc 1999;74(9):862–9.
85. Arquizan C, Coste J, Touboul PJ, et al. Is patent foramen ovale a family trait? A transcranial Doppler sonographic study. Stroke 2001;32(7):1563–6.
86. Seib G. Incidence of the patent foramen ovale cordis in adult American whites and American negroes. Am J Anat 1934;55:511–25.
87. Thompson T, Evans V. Paradoxical embolism. Q J Med 1930;23:135–52.
88. Hagen PT, Scholz DG, Edwards WD. Incidence and size of patent foramen ovale during the first 10 decades of life: an autopsy study of 965 normal hearts. Mayo Clin Proc 1984;59(1):17–20.
89. Di Tullio MR, Sacco RL, Sciacca RR, et al. Patent foramen ovale and the risk of ischemic stroke in a multiethnic population. J Am Coll Cardiol 2007;49(7): 797–802.
90. Pearson AC, Labovitz AJ, Tatineni S, et al. Superiority of transesophageal echocardiography in detecting cardiac source of embolism in patients with cerebral ischemia of uncertain etiology. J Am Coll Cardiol 1991;17(1):66–72.
91. Di Tullio M, Sacco RL, Venketasubramanian N, et al. Comparison of diagnostic techniques for the detection of a patent foramen ovale in stroke patients. Stroke 1993;24(7):1020–4.
92. Sloan MA, Alexandrov AV, Tegeler CH, et al. Assessment: transcranial Doppler ultrasonography: report of the Therapeutics and Technology Assessment Subcommittee of the American Academy of Neurology. Neurology 2004;62(9):1468–81.
93. Spencer MP, Moehring MA, Jesurum J, et al. Power m-mode transcranial Doppler for diagnosis of patent foramen ovale and assessing transcatheter closure. J Neuroimaging 2004;14(4):342–9.
94. Jesurum JT, Fuller CJ, Kim CJ, et al. Frequency of migraine headache relief following patent foramen ovale "closure" despite residual right-to-left shunt. Am J Cardiol 2008;102:916–20.
95. Jesurum JT, Fuller CJ, Moehring MA, et al. Unilateral versus bilateral middle cerebral artery detection of right-to-left shunt by power m-mode transcranial Doppler. J Neuroimaging 2009;19(3):235–41.
96. Del Sette M, Dinia L, Rizzi D, et al. Diagnosis of right-to-left shunt with transcranial Doppler and vertebrobasilar recording. Stroke 2007;38(8):2254–6.
97. Sacco RL, Ellenberg JH, Mohr JP, et al. Infarcts of undetermined cause: the NINCDS Stroke Data Bank. Ann Neurol 1989;25(4):382–90.
98. Cramer SC, Rordorf G, Maki JH, et al. Increased pelvic vein thrombi in cryptogenic stroke: results of the Paradoxical Emboli from Large Veins in Ischemic Stroke (PELVIS) Study. Stroke 2004;35(1):46–50.
99. Lechat P, Mas JL, Lascault G, et al. Prevalence of patent foramen ovale in patients with stroke. N Engl J Med 1988;318(18):1148–52.

100. Webster MW, Chancellor AM, Smith HJ, et al. Patent foramen ovale in young stroke patients. Lancet 1988;2(8601):11–2.
101. Cabanes L, Mas JL, Cohen A, et al. Atrial septal aneurysm and patent foramen ovale as risk factors for cryptogenic stroke in patients less than 55 years of age. A study using transesophageal echocardiography. Stroke 1993;24(12): 1865–73.
102. de Belder MA, Tourikis L, Leech G, et al. Risk of patent foramen ovale for thromboembolic events in all age groups. Am J Cardiol 1992;69(16):1316–20.
103. Di Tullio M, Sacco RL, Gopal A, et al. Patent foramen ovale as a risk factor for cryptogenic stroke. Ann Intern Med 1992;117(6):461–5.
104. Hausmann D, Mugge A, Becht I, et al. Diagnosis of patent foramen ovale by transesophageal echocardiography and association with cerebral and peripheral embolic events. Am J Cardiol 1992;70(6):668–72.
105. Overell JR, Bone I, Lees KR. Interatrial septal abnormalities and stroke: a meta-analysis of case-control studies. Neurology 2000;55(8):1172–9.
106. Handke M, Harloff A, Olschewski M, et al. Patent foramen ovale and cryptogenic stroke in older patients. N Engl J Med 2007;357(22):2262–8.
107. De Castro S, Cartoni D, Fiorelli M, et al. Morphological and functional characteristics of patent foramen ovale and their embolic implications. Stroke 2000; 31(10):2407–13.
108. Steiner MM, Di Tullio MR, Rundek T, et al. Patent foramen ovale size and embolic brain imaging findings among patients with ischemic stroke. Stroke 1998;29(5): 944–8.
109. Homma S, Sacco RL, Di Tullio MR, et al. Effect of medical treatment in stroke patients with patent foramen ovale: patent foramen ovale in Cryptogenic Stroke Study. Circulation 2002;105(22):2625–31.
110. Stone DA, Godard J, Corretti MC, et al. Patent foramen ovale: association between the degree of shunt by contrast transesophageal echocardiography and the risk of future ischemic neurologic events. Am Heart J 1996;131(1): 158–61.
111. Anzola GP, Zavarize P, Morandi E, et al. Transcranial Doppler and risk of recurrence in patients with stroke and patent foramen ovale. Eur J Neurol 2003;10(2): 129–35.
112. Hanley PC, Tajik AJ, Hynes JK, et al. Diagnosis and classification of atrial septal aneurysm by two-dimensional echocardiography: report of 80 consecutive cases. J Am Coll Cardiol 1985;6(6):1370–82.
113. Mas JL, Arquizan C, Lamy C, et al. Recurrent cerebrovascular events associated with patent foramen ovale, atrial septal aneurysm, or both. N Engl J Med 2001;345(24):1740–6.
114. Karttunen V, Hiltunen L, Rasi V, et al. Leiden and prothrombin gene mutation may predispose to paradoxical embolism in subjects with patent foramen ovale. Blood Coagul Fibrinolysis 2003;14(3):261–8.
115. Lichy C, Reuner KH, Buggle F, et al. Prothrombin G20210A mutation, but not factor V Leiden, is a risk factor in patients with persistent foramen ovale and otherwise unexplained cerebral ischemia. Cerebrovasc Dis 2003;16(1):83–7.
116. Pezzini A, Del Zotto E, Magoni M, et al. Inherited thrombophilic disorders in young adults with ischemic stroke and patent foramen ovale. Stroke 2003; 34(1):28–33.
117. Belvis R, Santamaria A, Marti-Fabregas J, et al. Patent foramen ovale and prothrombotic markers in young stroke patients. Blood Coagul Fibrinolysis 2007; 18(6):537–42.

118. Demirtas Tatlidede A, Oflazoglu B, Erten Celik S, et al. Prevalence of patent foramen ovale in patients with migraine. Agri 2007;19(4):39–42.
119. Wilmshurst PT, Pearson MJ, Nightingale S, et al. Inheritance of persistent foramen ovale and atrial septal defects and the relation to familial migraine with aura. Heart 2004;90(11):1315–20.
120. Anzola GP, Meneghetti G, Zanferrari C, et al. Is migraine associated with right-to-left shunt a separate disease? Results of the SAM Study. Cephalalgia 2008; 28(4):360–6.
121. Tembl J, Lago A, Sevilla T, et al. Migraine, patent foramen ovale and migraine triggers. J Headache Pain 2007;8(1):7–12.
122. Fukui PT, Goncalves TR, Strabelli CG, et al. Trigger factors in migraine patients. Arq Neuropsiquiatr 2008;66(3A):494–9.
123. Gori S, Morelli N, Fanucchi S, et al. The extent of right-to-left shunt fails to corre-late with severity of clinical picture in migraine with aura. Neurol Sci 2006;27(1): 14–7.
124. Rundek T, Elkind MS, Di Tullio MR, et al. Patent foramen ovale and migraine. A cross-sectional study from the Northern Manhattan Study (NOMAS). Circulation 2008;118(14):1419–24.
125. Sacco RL, Adams R, Albers G, et al. Guidelines for prevention of stroke in patients with ischemic stroke or transient ischemic attack: a statement for healthcare professionals from the American Heart Association/American Stroke Association Council on Stroke: co-sponsored by the Council on Cardiovascular Radiology and Intervention: the American Academy of Neurology affirms the value of this guideline. Circulation 2006;113(10):e409–49.
126. Slottow TL, Steinberg DH, Waksman R. Overview of the 2007 Food and Drug Administration Circulatory System Devices Panel meeting on patent foramen ovale closure devices. Circulation 2007;116(6):677–82.
127. Wilmshurst PT, Nightingale S, Walsh KP, et al. Effect on migraine of closure of cardiac right-to-left shunts to prevent recurrence of decompression illness or stroke or for haemodynamic reasons. Lancet 2000;356:1648–51.
128. Schwerzmann M, Wiher S, Nedeltchev K, et al. Percutaneous closure of patent foramen ovale reduces the frequency of migraine attacks. Neurology 2004; 62(8):1399–401.
129. Slavin L, Tobis JM, Rangarajan K, et al. Five-year experience with percutaneous closure of patent foramen ovale. Am J Cardiol 2007;99(9):1316–20.
130. Anzola GP, Frisoni GB, Morandi E, et al. Shunt-associated migraine responds favorably to atrial septal repair. A case-control study. Stroke 2006; 37(2):430–4.
131. Wood S. NOMAS: just a 2% overlap for PFO and migraine; St. Jude shuts down ESCAPE trial. theheart.org. Accessed October 22, 2008.
132. Sarens T, Herroelen L, Van Deyk K, et al. Patent foramen ovale closure and migraine: are we following the wrong pathway? J Neurol 2009;256(1):143–4.
133. Rodes-Cabau J, Molina C, Serrano-Munuera C, et al. Migraine with aura related to the percutaneous closure of an atrial septal defect. Catheter Cardiovasc In-terv 2003;60(4):540–2.
134. Lai DW, Saver JL, Araujo JA, et al. Pericarditis associated with nickel hypersen-sitivity to the Amplatzer occluder device: a case report. Catheter Cardiovasc Interv 2005;66(3):424–6.
135. Wertman B, Azarbal B, Riedl M, et al. Adverse events associated with nickel allergy in patients undergoing percutaneous atrial septal defect or patent foramen ovale closure. J Am Coll Cardiol 2006;47(6):1226–7.

136. Ries MW, Kampmann C, Rupprecht HJ, et al. Nickel release after implantation of the Amplatzer occluder. Am Heart J 2003;145(4):737–41.

137. Jesurum JT, Fuller CJ, Velez CA, et al. Migraineurs with patent foramen ovale have larger right-to-left shunt despite similar atrial septal features. J Headache Pain 2007;8(4):209–16.

138. Renz J, Jesurum JT, Fuller CJ, et al. Diagnosis of secondary source of right-to-left shunt with balloon occlusion of patent foramen ovale and power m-mode transcranial Doppler. JACC Cardiovasc Interv 2009;2(6):561–7.

139. Meissner I, Khandheria BK, Heit JA, et al. Patent foramen ovale: innocent or guilty? Evidence from a prospective population-based study. J Am Coll Cardiol 2006;47(2):440–5.

140. Silvestrini M, Baruffaldi R, Bartolini M, et al. Basilar and middle cerebral artery reactivity in patients with migraine. Headache 2004;44(1):29–34.

141. Shanoudy H, Soliman A, Raggi P, et al. Prevalence of patent foramen ovale and its contribution to hypoxemia in patients with obstructive sleep apnea. Chest 1998;113(1):91–6.

142. van der Kuy P-HM, Lohman JJHM. A quantification of the placebo response in migraine prophylaxis. Cephalalgia 2002;22:265–70.

143. Macedo A, Farre M, Banos JE. A meta-analysis of the placebo response in acute migraine and how this response may be influenced by some of the characteristics of clinical trials. Eur J Clin Pharmacol 2006;62(3):161–72.

144. Giardini A, Donti A, Formigari R, et al. Spontaneous large right-to-left shunt and migraine headache with aura are risk factors for recurrent stroke in patients with a patent foramen ovale. Int J Cardiol 2007;120(3):357–62.

145. Goldstein LB, Adams R, Alberts MJ, et al. Primary prevention of ischemic stroke: a guideline from the American Heart Association/American Stroke Association Stroke Council: cosponsored by the Atherosclerotic Peripheral Vascular Disease Interdisciplinary Working Group; Cardiovascular Nursing Council; Clinical Cardiology Council; Nutrition, Physical Activity, and Metabolism Council; and the Quality of Care and Outcomes Research Interdisciplinary Working Group: the American Academy of Neurology affirms the value of this guideline. Stroke 2006;37(6):1583–633.

146. Ridker PM, Cook NR, Lee IM, et al. A randomized trial of low-dose aspirin in the primary prevention of cardiovascular disease in women. N Engl J Med 2005;352(13):1293–304.

147. Lev EI, Patel RT, Maresh KJ, et al. Aspirin and clopidogrel drug response in patients undergoing percutaneous coronary intervention: the role of dual drug resistance. J Am Coll Cardiol 2006;47(1):27–33.

148. Qayyum R, Becker DM, Yanek LR, et al. Platelet inhibition by aspirin 81 and 325 mg/day in men versus women without clinically apparent cardiovascular disease. Am J Cardiol 2008;101(8):1359–63.

149. Law M, Morris JK, Jordan R, et al. Headaches and the treatment of blood pressure: results from a meta-analysis of 94 randomized placebo-controlled trials with 24,000 participants. Circulation 2005;112(15):2301–6.

150. Silberstein SD, Neto W, Schmitt J, et al. Topiramate in migraine prevention: results of a large controlled trial. Arch Neurol 2004;61(4):490–5.

151. Mathew NT, Loder EW. Evaluating the triptans. Am J Med 2005;118(Suppl 1): 28S–35S.

152. Smith T, Blumenthal H, Diamond M, et al. Sumatriptan/Naproxen sodium for migraine: efficacy, health related quality of life, and satisfaction outcomes. Headache 2007;47(5):683–92.

153. Azarbal B, Tobis J, Suh W, et al. Association of interatrial shunts and migraine headaches: impact of transcatheter closure. J Am Coll Cardiol 2005;45(4): 489–92.
154. Dubiel M, Bruch L, Schmehl I, et al. Migraine headache relief after percutaneous transcatheter closure of interatrial communications. J Interv Cardiol 2008;21(1): 32–7.
155. Shaygannejad V, Janghorbani M, Ghorbani A, et al. Comparison of the effect of topiramate and sodium valporate in migraine prevention: a randomized blinded crossover study. Headache 2006;46(4):642–8.
156. Brandes JL, Kudrow D, Stark SR, et al. Sumatriptan-naproxen for acute treatment of migraine: a randomized trial. JAMA 2007;297(13):1443–54.

Emerging Inflammatory Biomarkers with Acute Stroke

Theresa M. Wadas, PhD(c), RN, FNP-BC, ACNP-BC, CCRN[a,b,*]

KEYWORDS

• Biomarker • Inflammation • Stroke • Cerebral • Ischemia

Stroke remains the third leading cause of death in the United States and is a significant public health burden, affecting 795,000 individuals annually with direct and indirect expenditures in 2009 exceeding \$68 billion.[1] Although the past decade heralded exciting developments in neuroimaging, particularly the identification of the ischemic penumbra with diffusion/perfusion MRI and the use of high-speed CT,[2] timely and accurate diagnosis of acute stroke remains a significant challenge. One in five Medicare stroke hospitalizations receives an "ill-defined" diagnosis, suggesting that a disturbing proportion of patients may not receive adequate treatment.[3]

The diagnosis of stroke is based on history and clinical examination of the patient supplemented by accurate interpretation of neuroimaging. Neuroimaging is used to distinguish between hemorrhagic and ischemic stroke. Neuroimaging can be difficult, however, because CT generally is insensitive to cerebral ischemia and the scan may be normal following the onset of ischemia. Additionally, although MRI is more sensitive than CT for cerebral ischemia, MRI is time consuming, possibly delaying acute stroke treatment, may be contraindicated in select patients, and may not be readily available.[4] Thus, the ability to identify stroke patients rapidly by using a biologic biomarker would be highly beneficial in facilitating diagnosis and therapeutic interventions, preventing adverse clinical outcomes, and decreasing health care costs.

A biomarker is "a characteristic that is objectively measured and evaluated as an indicator of normal biologic processes, pathogenic processes, or pharmacologic response to a therapeutic intervention."[5] Biologic biomarkers usually are measured from body fluids such as blood, urine, or tissue samples. The sensitivity of a biomarker refers to its ability to detect disease when the disease is present.[6] The specificity of a biomarker refers to its ability to exclude the disease when the disease is not

[a] Adult Acute Nurse Practitioner Program, School of Nursing, University of Alabama at Birmingham, NB 544, 1530 3rd Avenue South, Birmingham, Alabama 35294-1210, USA
[b] College of Nursing, University of Arizona, 1305 N. Martin, Tucson, AZ 85721-0203, USA
* Adult Acute Nurse Practitioner Program, School of Nursing, University of Alabama at Birmingham, NB 544, 1530 3rd Avenue South, Birmingham, Alabama 35294-1210.
E-mail address: twadas@uab.edu

Crit Care Nurs Clin N Am 21 (2009) 493–505
doi:10.1016/j.ccell.2009.07.010
0899-5885/09/\$ – see front matter © 2009 Elsevier Inc. All rights reserved.

present.[6] The development of reference standard biologic biomarkers for diagnosing and evaluating stroke is problematic, however, because of the complexity of stroke physiology, the heterogeneity of stroke, and the presence of the blood–brain barrier.[7]

In general, the term "stroke" refers to an umbrella of conditions that result from compromised blood flow or hemorrhage of blood vessels supplying the brain.[8] Stroke therefore is categorized broadly as either hemorrhagic or ischemic, with varying degrees of hemorrhagic transformation (HT) or permeability of the blood–brain barrier. Moreover, many patients who have acute stroke first present not to the hospital but rather to a primary care practitioner, a paramedic, or the triage nurse of an urgent care clinic. In a 2002 survey conducted by the Center for Disease Control, 21% of the counties in the United States did not have a hospital, 31% lacked a hospital with an emergency department, and 77% did not have a hospital with neurologic services.[9] These challenges have led researchers to examine physiologic mechanisms that may serve as potential biomarkers for the diagnosis and evaluation of acute stroke.

Inflammation is one physiologic mechanism that has been studied extensively in relation to stroke. This article presents a review of emerging inflammatory biomarkers of acute stroke and discusses (1) the physiologic basis of inflammation and stroke, (2) inflammatory biomarkers associated with acute stroke, and (3) the challenges of using inflammatory biomarkers to diagnose acute stroke.

THE PHYSIOLOGIC BASIS OF INFLAMMATION AND STROKE

During the past several decades, much of what has become known about inflammatory processes associated with stroke has been derived from animal models of ischemic stroke. This knowledge is the focus of this discussion. Cessation of cerebral blood flow or decreased blood flow below critical levels results in various cellular mechanisms that are characterized by the influx of peripheral leukocytes into the cerebral parenchyma and the activation of microglia. These cellular events are accompanied by changes in the cerebral microvasculature, which include energy failure, metabolism abnormalities, and intra- and extracellular membrane abnormalities, resulting in the release of glutamate and other excitatory and inhibitory amino acids such as glycine and γ-aminobutyric acid (GABA).[10] Neurons, astrocytes, microglia, and endothelial cells are activated in response to cerebral ischemia with subsequent release of various inflammatory mediators.

Cytokines are inflammatory mediators that are glycoproteins and are able to interact among themselves and with other cell types. Interleukin (IL) 1β, IL-6, and tissue necrosis factor alpha (TNF-α) are cytokines that have an important role in this inflammatory response. The activation of IL-1β and TNF-α initiates this inflammatory process, which occurs early in cerebral ischemia and is transient. IL-1β and TNF-α induce a secondary response that is more lasting and is mediated by IL-6 and IL-8.[11,12]

Cytokines also stimulate the release of adhesion molecules. Adhesion molecules include selectins, the superfamily of immunoglobulins, and integrins, which through their coordinated efforts contribute to leukocyte activation, recruitment, and aggregation in the cerebral microvasculature.[11–13] Selectins (L-selectin, E-selectin, and P-selectin) are glycoproteins that are useful in the interaction between leukocyte endothelial cells, platelets, leukocytes, and lymphocytes.[11,12] Their cellular interactions are crucial for inflammatory and thrombotic processes. L-selectin and E-selectin are found on leukocytes and endothelial cells; P selectins are found on both platelets and endothelial cells. The primary molecules of the superfamily of immunoglobulins include intercellular adhesion molecule type 1 (ICAM-1) and vascular cell adhesion molecule type 1 (VCAM-1), which participate in the acute phase of cerebral ischemia.[11,12]

The integrins participate in intercellular adhesion and bind to extracellular matrix components mediated by other groups of adhesions. In the brain, integrins connect the cells that comprise the blood–brain barrier and thus are crucial for the integrity of the cerebral microvasculature.[11,12] The resulting inflammatory response includes the recruitment of polymorphonuclear (PMN) leukocytes and its adhesion to the vascular wall, resulting in obstruction of the microvasculature.[14–16]

The hallmark features of inflammation associated with ischemic stroke are neuron loss, cerebral edema, and the presence of PMN leukocytes with cellular necrosis and tissue infarction as the end result.[11,12] Reperfusion of the occluded vessel either through collateral circulation or spontaneous or therapeutic means results in the generation of reactive oxygen species (ROS).[8,12,14] ROS can stimulate ischemic cells to secrete inflammatory cytokines and chemokines that lead to increased numbers of inflammatory cells, such as cell adhesion molecules, in the cerebral vasculature and systemically. These inflammatory cells then release various cytotoxic substances including more cytokines, matrix metalloproteinases (MMPs), nitric oxide (NO), and more ROS.[8,12,14]

MMPs are a family of proteolytic enzymes that are responsible for extracellular matrix remodeling. MMP-2 and MMP-9 as well as NO and ROS have been implicated in further cellular damage and may affect the blood–brain barrier.[9,17] Disruption of the blood–brain barrier may potentiate further brain tissue injury and contribute to secondary ischemic brain injury by allowing various substances and blood to enter the brain.[11,12] Secondary damage also may result from cerebral edema, hypoperfusion or hemodynamic instability, and postischemic inflammation.[12] Secondary damage may be particularly pronounced when blocked vessels become open and a massive influx of ROS and leukocytes enters the injured brain, resulting in reperfusion injury.[11,12] **Fig. 1** illustrates the inflammatory mechanisms within the cerebral microvasculature as a result of blood flow interruption. **Fig. 2** summarizes the inflammation process following ischemic stroke.

INFLAMMATORY BIOMARKERS AND STROKE

From the inflammatory cascade, several inflammatory biomarkers of cerebral ischemia and infarct have been proposed in the acute phase to (1) diagnose stroke, (2) predict the evolution of stroke, and (3) predict the development of HT either spontaneously or after therapeutic intervention. In addition, several inflammatory biomarkers have emerged from various preliminary studies as potential candidates and remain the subject of ongoing research, particularly with a multiple-biomarker strategy and in combination with neuroimaging.

INFLAMMATORY MARKERS ASSOCIATED WITH THE DIAGNOSIS OF STROKE

The evaluation and selection of candidate biomarkers for the diagnosis of stroke was tested recently with 26 biomarkers, including biomarkers of glial activation (protein S-100 beta), inflammation (MMP-9 and VCAM-1), and other cellular processes, such as coagulation and fibrinolysis. Of the biomarkers evaluated in 65 patients suspected of having experienced stroke and 157 control patients, four biomarkers were highly correlated with stroke (with a sensitivity and specificity of 90% for predicting stroke): protein S-100 beta, MMP-9, VCAM-1, and von Willebrand factor.[18]

The same group of researchers later evaluated a five-biomarker panel (protein S-100 beta, B-type neurotrophic growth factor, von Willebrand factor, MMP-9, and monocyte chemotactic protein) in 214 healthy controls and 221 patients who had

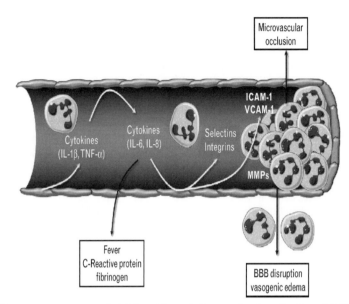

Fig. 1. Inflammatory response is initiated by cytokine activation (IL-1β and TNF-α). These cytokines start a second inflammatory response, activating IL-6 and IL-8, which mediate the development of acute-phase reactants (fever, C-reactive protein, and fibrinogen) and the release of cell adhesion molecules, causing microvascular occlusion. Finally, MMPs help in the migration of leukocyte and blood–brain barrier (BBB) disruption, leading to vascular edema. (*From* Rodrigues-Yanez M, Castillo J. Role of inflammatory markers in brain ischemia. Curr Opin Neurol 2008;21(3):354; with permission.)

stroke (including 122 patients diagnosed with ischemic stroke). By using a panel algorithm in which three or more biomarker values were scored as positive, this five-biomarker panel provided a sensitivity of 93% and a specificity of 93% for the diagnosis of ischemic and hemorrhagic stroke within the first 6 hours after onset.[19]

A more recent multicenter trial at 17 different sites evaluated point-of-care testing with a four-biomarker panel (MMP-9, protein S100 beta, D dimer, and brain natriuretic protein) in 1146 patients presenting with neurologic symptoms suspicious of stroke. An additional cohort of 343 patients also was enrolled to validate the multiple-biomarker approach. A diagnostic tool that incorporated the biomarker values into one composite score was found to be sensitive for acute cerebral ischemia. The results indicated a sensitivity of 86% for detecting all strokes and a sensitivity of 94% for detecting hemorrhagic stroke.[7] These results were reproducible in the separate validation cohort. Although the diagnostic accuracy of this biomarker panel clearly is not ideal, because several of these biomarkers can be elevated in various pathologic conditions, this study is significant because demonstrates the feasibility of incorporating a point-of-care biomarker algorithm with available clinical data and neuroimaging to aid in the early identification of stroke.

INFLAMMATORY BIOMARKERS ASSOCIATED WITH THE PREDICTION OF THE EVOLUTION OF STROKE

In addition to diagnosing stroke, the evolution of stroke is also of interest, particularly when timely therapeutic interventions may be able to save brain tissue at risk. Optimistic developments have occurred with high-speed CT, perfusion-weighted (PWI)

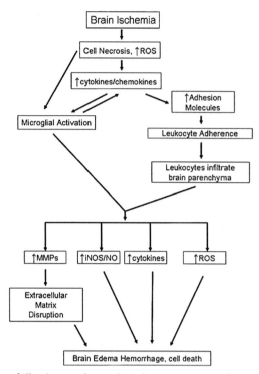

Fig. 2. Inflammation following stroke. Brain ischemia triggers inflammatory responses resulting from the presence of necrotic cells, the generation of ROS, and the production of inflammatory cytokines even within neurons. These initiators lead to microglial activation that produces more cytokines, causing upregulation of adhesion molecules in the cerebral vasculature. Chemokines lead to inflammatory cell chemotaxis to ischemic brain. Adhesion molecules mediate adhesion of circulating leukocytes to vascular endothelia and infiltration into the brain parenchyma. Once in the brain, activated leukocytes and microglia produced a variety of inflammable mediators such as MMPs, inducible nitric oxide synthase (iNOS), which generates NO, cytokines, and more ROS, which lead to brain edema, hemorrhage and ultimately, cell death. MMPs are thought to mediate extracellular matrix disruption, a key event in brain edema and hemorrhage. (*From* Wang Q, Tang XN, Yenari MA. The inflammatory response in stroke. J Neuroimmunol 2007;184(1–2):53; with permission.)

and diffusion-weighted (DWI) MRI techniques, and inflammatory biomarkers to predict and evaluate the evolution of stroke. DWI and PWI MRI techniques make it possible to study cellular injury such as the entry of intracellular water as the earliest marker of cerebral ischemia and altered cerebral perfusion during hyperacute stroke.[2] A recent preliminary study investigated the correlation of inflammatory biomarkers and PWI and DWI of lesions and studied this relationship further in regards to the evolution cerebral infarct. In 16 patients who had middle cerebral artery stroke, MMP-2, MMP-9, IL-6, IL-8, TNF-α, and ICAM-1 were measured upon presentation (less than 6 hours after onset). Findings revealed that MMP-9 was the only predictor of infarct volume measured as a DWI lesion. Additional findings demonstrated that the extent of hypoperfused brain was associated with the release of proinflammatory cytokine releases (TNF-α and IL-6) over the next few hours. Furthermore, ICAM-1, which was measured at 12- and 24-hour time points correlated with the final DWI lesions measured at day 5 to day 7.[20] Although the sample size was small, these preliminary findings suggest a close relationship between the hypoperfused brain and proinflammatory cytokine release and between tissue destruction and MMP-9, suggesting that endothelial damage may participate in the enlargement of ischemic lesions.

Another study was conducted on 271 patients who had hemispheric ischemic stroke of less than 24 hours' evolution. The early signs of cerebral ischemia were classified as hypodensity with and without mass effect. Findings demonstrated that increased levels of excitotoxicity biomarkers (glutamate), inflammatory biomarkers (TNF-α and IL-6), and the rupture of the blood–brain barrier (MMP-9) were associated with higher degrees of cerebral edema.[17]

Findings of elevated inflammatory biomarkers during the evolution of stroke raise the question whether treatment directed at inhibition of the inflammatory response during this critical time could save cerebral tissue at risk and minimize cerebral ischemia, infarct, and edema. **Fig. 3** summarizes the inflammatory markers that have been investigated in the evolution of stroke.

INFLAMMATORY BIOMARKERS ASSOCIATED WITH HEMORRHAGIC TRANSFORMATION

HT is classified as hemorrhagic infarction, characterized by petechial hemorrhage primarily affecting the ischemic zone, or parenchymal hematoma, characterized by discrete masses of blood beginning in the ischemic zone with mass effect that may extend to the ventricle.[21] Although the development of HT can occur as part of the natural evolution of cerebral ischemia, predicting its development is of significance, particularly in patients who may benefit from thrombolytic therapy.

Forty-fifty percent of patients who suffer a thrombolytic stroke do not recanalize or do so too late, and 6% to 15% develop HT, with high mortality rates.[22] Tissue plasminogen activator (tPA) increases the possibility of HT by degrading the integrity of the extracellular matrix and increases the risk of neurovascular cell death, blood–brain barrier leakage, edema, and hemorrhage.[23,24] Additionally, hypertension, use of anticoagulants, age, hyperglycemia, the presence of early signs of ischemia on CT, and extension of the cerebral infarct have been associated with HT.[17,24]

HT can be viewed as a result of the inflammatory process following ischemic injury. Following middle cerebral artery occlusion, integrin expression with endothelial cells and astrocytes of the microvasculature is lost, ultimately affecting the basal lamina.

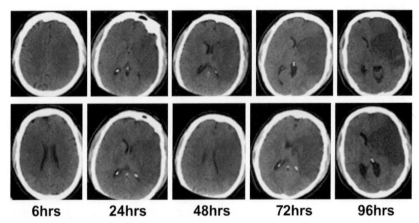

6hrs   24hrs   48hrs   72hrs   96hrs

Fig. 3. Association of inflammatory biomarkers with onset and first 96hrs of stroke. 6hrs, 24hrs, 48hrs, 72hrs and 96hrs post infarct.

The loss of integrity of the endothelial basal lamina of the cerebral microcirculation is the primary cause of HT following cerebral ischemia.[21,25] **Fig. 4** illustrates effects of ischemia on the microvascular integrity, contributing to HT.

Several studies in patients who suffered ischemic stroke have demonstrated the association between high levels of MMP-9 and the risk of developing HT, with and without the use of thrombolytic therapy.[26,27] Plasma levels of MMP-9 were found to be three times higher in patients who had HT.[27] Plasma MMP-9 levels greater than 140 ng/mL independently predicted the development of HT in ischemic patients with a sensitivity of 87% and a specificity of 90%.[27] In a similar study of patients who had cardioembolic stroke who had received thrombolytic therapy, plasma MMP-9 levels greater than 191.3 ng/mL predicted the development of HT with a sensitivity of 100% and specificity of 78%.[26] **Fig. 5** illustrates the development of HT and the associated inflammatory biomarkers after tPA infusion.

Studies also have shown that the administration of an MMP inhibitor reduces the incidence and severity of HT induced by thrombolytic therapy.[28,29] These results are promising. In the future, as the therapeutic time window may be extended beyond 3 hours, the administration of thrombolytic therapy with an MMP inhibitor may decrease the incidence of HT and provide further therapeutic benefit.[23] Moreover, stroke biomarker profiling may be able to indicate the best reperfusion strategy for individual patients.

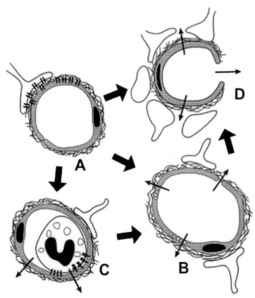

Fig. 4. Effects of ischemia on microvascular integrity. (*A*) Normal cerebral microvessel. Endothelial cells and astrocytes are attached to the matrix by adhesion receptors. The endothelial blood–brain barrier is intact. (*B*) Following focal ischemia, there is an increase in endothelial cell permeability, (*C*) expression of leukocyte adhesion receptors in postcapillary venules, mediating leukocyte adhesion and transmigration which affect permeability, and (*D*) breakdown of basal lamina with loss of astrocyte and endothelial cell contacts and increased permeability to cell (eg, erythrocytes). (*From* Del Zoppo GJ, Hallenbeck JM. Advances in the vascular pathophysiology of ischemic stroke. Thromb Res 2000;98(3):V75; with permission.)

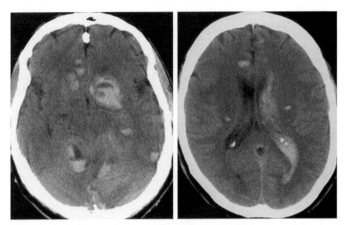

Fig. 5. Post-thrombolytic hemorrhage is illustrated via CT scan and is associated with increased plasma levels of MMP-9.

CHALLENGES IN THE DEVELOPMENT OF INFLAMMATORY BIOMARKERS

The single greatest challenge in the development of stroke biomarkers is the lack of a reference standard as a diagnostic or prognostic tool for stroke.[30] As previously stated, biologic biomarkers for diagnosing and evaluating stroke are problematic because of the complexity of stroke physiology, the heterogeneity of stroke, and the presence of the blood–brain barrier.[7] Thus, the standard reference for the diagnosis of stroke remains the clinical decision by an expert clinician, even in the absence of any hard end point or objective data.

Before inflammatory biomarkers or other stroke biomarkers can be incorporated into clinical practice, the biochemical and clinical characteristics must be established for each biomarker, and its value as a clinical tool must be established by appropriate validity studies. New clinical biomarkers, whether representing inflammation or another physiologic process associated with stroke, are of clinical value only if they are accurate, reproducible, acceptable to the patient, inexpensive, and easy to interpret by the health care team and provide information that has a high degree of sensitivity and specificity (**Table 1**).[6]

Generally, the desired properties of biomarkers vary with their intended purpose. For the diagnosis of acute stroke, the ideal biomarker includes all the features mentioned as well as rapid sustained elevation, a high level of sensitivity, release that is proportional to the acute event, and assay features that permit point-of-care testing.[6] Although inflammatory biomarkers have yet to meet all these characteristics and criteria, they do provide additive information, particularly when added to current clinical tools such as history, clinical examination, and neuroimaging. For this reason, multiple-biomarker strategies are used in stroke research to allow each biomarker to provide independent and additive information for its intended clinical application.[31] The multiple-biomarker approach can improve the predictive accuracy of disease states. **Fig. 6** provides a list of the various biomarkers and their physiologic mechanisms that can be used in a multiple-biomarker strategy to guide future stroke biomarker research and to augment current clinical tools.

An additional challenge associated with the use of inflammatory biomarkers for diagnosis of stroke is that stroke often does not occur in isolation but is associated with a myriad of comorbidities such as coronary artery disease, hypertension,

Table 1
Desirable features of biomarkers

All Biomarkers	Diagnostic Biomarkers	Prognostic/Treatment Biomarkers
General features	High stroke specificity	Known reference limits
Measures a specific pathology	Not present in normal serum	Adds to known prognostic index
Adds to clinical assessment	Zero baseline, immediate release with early detection	Change in marker alters management
Acceptable to patient		Affects choice of drug
Linear relation between change in marker and change in pathology	Permits a long-time window for diagnosis, but less than 24 hours	Changes dose of drug
Stable product	Release proportionate to injury size	Indicates tolerance
Applicable to men and women, different ages, different ethnicities	Convenience for point-of-care testing	Used for monitoring progression of disease
Replicated in multiple studies	Rapid results	Trajectory of marker correlates with disease progression
Assay measurement features	No special sample preparation needed	"Rule out" strategy with high specificity more important to avoid mislabeling asymptomatic cases.
Internationally standardized	Inexpensive	Cost effective
Accuracy	Readily available	
Precision	Diagnostic cutoff well defined and accepted	
Assay application features	Change management, triage, or specific treatment	
High sensitivity and specificity	"Rule out" strategy with high sensitivity more important to avoid missing disease	
	Cost effective	

Data from Vasan RS. Biomarkers of cardiovascular disease: molecular basis and practical considerations. Circulation 2006;113(199):2337.

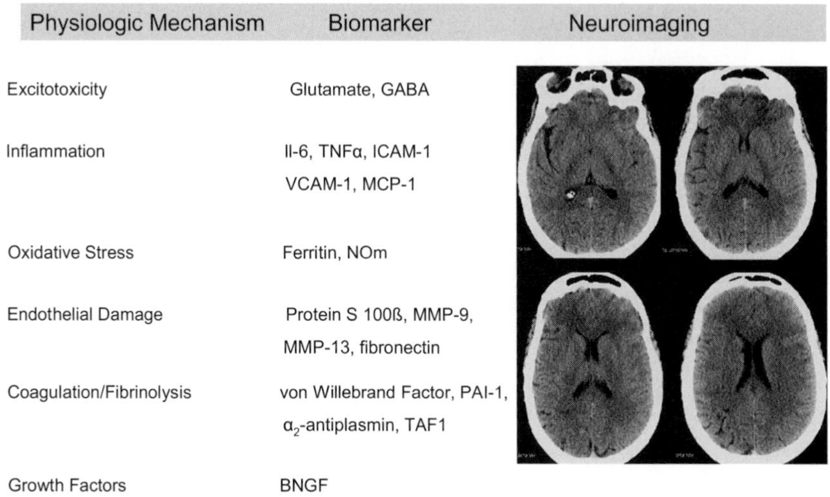

Physiologic Mechanism	Biomarker	Neuroimaging
Excitotoxicity	Glutamate, GABA	
Inflammation	Il-6, TNFα, ICAM-1 VCAM-1, MCP-1	
Oxidative Stress	Ferritin, NOm	
Endothelial Damage	Protein S 100ß, MMP-9, MMP-13, fibronectin	
Coagulation/Fibrinolysis	von Willebrand Factor, PAI-1, α_2-antiplasmin, TAF1	
Growth Factors	BNGF	

Fig. 6. The physiologic mechanism and associated biomarkers that may be used with neuroimaging. BNGF, B-type neurotrophic growth factor; MCP, monocyte chemotactic protein; Nom, nitric oxide metabolites; PAI-1, plasminogen activator inhibitor; TAF1, thrombin-activated fibrinolysis inhibitor.

Table 2
Five phases of biomarker development from discovery to delivery. "Content validity" refers to the degree to which the biomarker represents the biologic phenomenon studied (eg, MMP-9 represents BBB disruption). "Construct validity" refers to establishing that the biomarker is measuring the aspect of disease (some conceptual construct of theory) that investigators want to measure (eg, inflammation); therefore, one should establish whether serum IL-6 and TNF-α relate to inflammation. "Criterion validity" refers to how well the biomarker identifies the disease state (eg, how well MMP-9 predicts hemorrhagic transformation) when compared with a reference standard (measured in terms of sensitivity and specificity).

Phases:	Phase 1 Preclinical Exploratory	Phase 2 Clinical Characterization & Assay Validation	Phase 3 Clinical Association: Retrospective Repository Studies	Phase 4 Clinical Association: Prospective Screening Studies	Phase 5 Disease Control
Objective	Target Biomarker identification, Feasibility	Study assay in people with & without disease	Case-control studies using repository specimens	Longitudinal studies to predict disease	Clinical use
Site	Biomarker Development Lab	Biomarker Validation Lab	Clinical Epidemiologic Centers	Cohort Studies	Community
Design	Cross-sectional	Cross-sectional	Case-control	Prospective	RCT
Sample Size	Small	Small	Modest	Medium	Large
Validity	Content & construct validity	Criterion validity	Predictive validity	Efficacy of strategy	Effectiveness
Result	Assay precision reliability sensitivity	Reference limits, intra-individual variation	Screening characteristics, true & false + rates	ROC analyses	No.-needed-to screen/treat

Abbreviation: RCT, randomized controlled trial.
Data from Vassan RS. Biomarkers of cardiovascular disease: Molecular basis and practical considerations. Circulation. 2006;113:2348.

diabetes mellitus, and obesity, all of which may influence an individual's inflammatory state. The blood–brain barrier also affects biomarkers. Biomarkers may be elevated from the initial cerebral insult but may not be evident in the plasma because of the blood–brain barrier, a particular challenge when the critical time for administration of thrombolytics is within 3 hours of stroke onset. Finally, the ultimate goal of stroke biomarker research is to translate these biomarkers to the cellular pathways that characterize the disease process and to use these biochemical data to aid in diagnosis and management. Such an endeavor is no easy feat and clearly relies on the expertise of and the collaborative efforts among clinical investigators, biochemists, bioinformatics specialists, and all members of the health care team across services and departments. **Table 2** outlines the five phases of biomarker development from discovery to clinical use and illustrates the current status of stroke biomarker research.

SUMMARY

Despite newer neuroimaging techniques, timely and accurate diagnosis of acute stroke remains a significant challenge. Inflammatory mechanisms associated with ischemic stroke suggest that various inflammatory biomarkers may serve as an additional clinical tool for diagnosing stroke, predicting the evolution of stroke, and predicting HT. Challenges in biomarker research must be overcome, however, before the widespread adoption of biomarkers in clinical practice can be recommended.

Stroke physiology is complex and is complicated further by issues of stroke heterogeneity, the blood–brain barrier, and other inflammatory disease states. In the absence of a reference standard, comparative analyses are difficult. Nevertheless, emerging inflammatory biomarkers demonstrate considerable promise, particularly as part of a multiple biomarker strategy; if the use of these biomarkers proves successful, significant improvements in diagnosis, clinical management, and outcomes may be realized. Research in biomarkers for acute stroke will remain an active area of investigation and has the potential to make a substantial impact on the overall burden of stroke, both in the United States and worldwide.

REFERENCES

1. Lloyd-Jones D, Adams HP, Carnethon M, et al. American Heart Association Statistics Committee and Stroke Statistics Subcommittee. Heart disease and stroke statistics–2009 update. A report from the American Heart Association Statistics Committee and Stroke Statistics Subcommittee. Circulation 2009;119: e51–66.
2. Gonzalez RG. Imaging guided acute ischemic stroke therapy: from "time to brain" to "physiology is brain". AJNR Am J Neuroradiol 2006;27(4):728–35.
3. McGruder HF, Croft JB, Zheng ZJ. Characteristics of an "ill defined" diagnosis for stroke: opportunities for improvement. Stroke 2006;37(3):781–9.
4. Whiteley W, Tsend M, Sandercock P. Blood biomarkers in the diagnosis of ischemic stroke: a systematic review. Stroke 2008;39(10):2902–9.
5. Atkinson AJ, Colburn WA, DeGruttola VG, et al. Biomarkers Definitions Working Group. Biomarkers and surrogate endpoints: preferred definitions and conceptual framework. Clin Pharmacol Ther 2001;69(3):89–95.
6. Vasan RS. Biomarkers of cardiovascular disease: molecular basis and practical considerations. Circulation 2006;113(19):2335–62.
7. Laskowitz DT, Kasner SE, Saver J, et al. Brain Study Group. Clinical usefulness of a biomarker-based diagnostic test for acute stroke. The Biomarker Rapid Assessment in Ischemic Injury (BRAIN) Study. Stroke 2009;40(1):1–11.

8. Lo EH, Dalkara T, Moskowitz MA. Mechanisms, challenge, and opportunities in stroke. Nat Rev Neurosci 2003;4(5):399–415.
9. Department of Health and Human Services, Centers for Disease Control and Prevention. First-ever county level report on stroke hospitalizations. CDC Press Release. Available at: http://www.cdc.gov/media/pressrel/2008/r0803.htm; March 28, 2008. Accessed November 27, 2008.
10. Gusev E, Skvortsova VI. Brain ischemia. New York: Plenum Publishers; 2003. p. 39–93.
11. Huang J, Urvashi M, Upadhyay BS, et al. Inflammation in stroke and focal cerebral ischemia. Surg Neurol 2006;66(3):232–45.
12. Wang Q, Tang XN, Yenari MA. The inflammatory response in stroke. J Neuroimmunol 2007;184(1–2):53–68.
13. Rodrigues-Yanez M, Castillo J. Role of inflammatory markers in brain ischemia. Curr Opin Neurol 2008;21(3):353–7.
14. Zheng Z, Yenari M. Post-ischemic inflammation: molecular mechanisms and therapeutic implications. Neurol Res 2004;26(8):884–92.
15. Del Zoppo GJ, Schmid-Schonbein GW, Mori E, et al. Polymorphonuclear leukocytes occlude capillaries following middle cerebral artery occlusion and reperfusion in baboons. Stroke 1991;22(10):1276–83.
16. Del Zoppo GJ. Microvascular responses to cerebral ischemia/inflammation. Ann N Y Acad Sci 1997;823:132–47.
17. Castillo J, Rodriguez I. Biochemical changes and inflammatory response as markers for brain ischemia: molecular markers of diagnostic utility and prognosis in human clinical practice. Cerebrovasc Dis 2004;17(Suppl 1):7–18.
18. Lynch JR, Blessing R, White WD, et al. Novel diagnostic test for acute stroke. Stroke 2004;35(1):57–63.
19. Reynolds MA, Kirchick HJ, Dahlen JR, et al. Early biomarkers of stroke. Clin Chem 2003;49(10):1733–9.
20. Montaner J, Rovira A, Mollina CA, et al. Plasmatic level of neuroinflammatory markers predict the extent of diffusion-weighted image lesions in hyperacute stroke. J Cereb Blood Flow Metab 2003;23(12):1403–7.
21. Del Zoppo GJ, Hallenbeck JM. Advances in the vascular pathophysiology of ischemic stroke. Thromb Res 2000;98(3):V73–81.
22. Montaner J. Stroke biomarkers: can they help us to guide stroke thrombolysis? Drug News Perspect 2006;19(9):523–32.
23. Montaner J, Molina CA, Monasterio J, et al. Matrix metalloproteinase-9 pretreatment level predicts intracranial hemorrhagic complications after thrombolysis in human stroke. Circulation 2003;107(4):598–603.
24. The NINDS t-PA Stroke Study Group. Intracerebral hemorrhage after intravenous t-PA therapy for ischemic stroke. Stroke 1997;28(11):2109–18.
25. Hamann GF, Okada Y, Fitridge R, et al. Microvascular basal lamina antigens disappear during cerebral ischemia and reperfusion. Stroke 1995;26(11):2120–6.
26. Montaner J, Alvariz-Sabin J, Molina CA, et al. Matrix metalloproteinase expression is related to hemorrhagic transformation after cardioembolic stroke. Stroke 2001;32(12):2762–7.
27. Castellanos M, Leira R, Serena J, et al. Plasma metalloproteinase-9 concentration predicts hemorrhage transformation in acute ischemic stroke. Stroke 2003;34(1):40–6.
28. Lapchak PA, Chapman D, Zivin JA. Metalloproteinase inhibition reduced thrombolytic (tissue plasminogen activation)-induced hemorrhage after thromboembolic stroke. Stroke 2000;31(12):3034–40.

29. Sumii T, Lo EH. Involvement of matrix metalloproteinase in thrombolysis-associated hemorrhagic transformation after embolic focal ischemia in rats. Stroke 2002;33(3):831–6.
30. Jensen MB, Chacon MR, Sattin JA, et al. The promise and potential pitfalls of serum biomarkers for ischemic stroke and transient ischemic attack. Neurologist 2008;14(4):243–6.
31. Laskowitz DT, Blessing R, Floyd J, et al. Panel of biomarkers predict stroke [abstract]. Ann N Y Acad Sci 2005;1053:30.

Glycemic Control in the Diabetic Patient After Stroke

Loretta T. Lee, RN, MSN, CRNP

KEYWORDS

• Diabetes • Stroke • Hyperglycemia • Glycemic control

Hyperglycemia is a common problem in the diabetic patient after an acute stroke. All diabetic patients are at increased risk of developing hyperglycemia or abnormally high concentrations of glucose in the blood stream after an acute stroke. Elevations in serum glucose can be due to contributing factors such as advanced age, obesity, physiologic stress, and the simple implementation of nutritional support. Maintaining therapeutic blood glucose levels in diabetics during extreme physiologic stress can present extreme challenges. Persistent states of hyperglycemia can have a devastating impact on the ischemic brain and rapidly increase brain infarct size, posing a serious threat to neurologic outcome in acute stroke.[1] Therefore, reasonably tight, yet therapeutic, control of glycemia in the diabetic stroke patient must be a priority.

The purpose of this article is to evaluate strategies for lowering glycemia, to improve neurologic outcome in acute stroke patients, and define the critical role of nurses in prevention or control of hyperglycemia.

EPIDEMIOLOGY

A careful review of the literature dating back to 2000 reveals alarming health statistics for diabetic patients. In the year 2000, it was estimated that 17.7 million people in the United States suffered from diabetes. China was estimated to have 20.8 million sufferers, and India 31.7 million sufferers. By the year 2010, it is believed that these alarming statistics will increase even more; it is estimated that there will be 30.3 million diabetics in the United States, 42.3 million in China and 79.4 million in India.[2]

In 2007, 8% of the US population had received a diagnosis of diabetes.[3] This 8% was an increase of 13.5% since 2005. In the year 1998, only about 50% of diabetics were aware of their diabetes. Despite these statistics, diabetes, and the devastating complications of hyperglycemia, continues to increase.

Department of Adult/Acute Health, Chronic Care and Foundations, UAB University of Alabama School of Nursing, NB 542 1530 3rd Avenue South, Birmingham, AL 35294-1210, USA
E-mail address: llee@uab.edu

Crit Care Nurs Clin N Am 21 (2009) 507–515
doi:10.1016/j.ccell.2009.08.002
0899-5885/09/$ – see front matter © 2009 Elsevier Inc. All rights reserved.
ccnursing.theclinics.com

Diabetes is a known risk factor for stroke.[4,5] Almost 70% of people with diabetes die from stroke or heart disease.[6] A review of death certificates of people 65 years and older in the United States for the year 2004 revealed that stroke was reported as the cause of death in 16% of reported diabetes-related cases.[7] Today, stroke does not generally result in immediate death, and mortality is significantly correlated with the type of stroke. Over 4 million stroke survivors reside in the United States today.[8] Of these survivors, a large percentage require institutionalization because of their neurologic disabilities. In instances in which one survives a stroke, the physiologic and psychological changes for these patients can be devastating. Yet stroke is preventable, and among other primary prevention measures, strict glycemic control may alter the fate of diabetic stroke patients otherwise destined for a poor prognosis.

Diabetes is a major concern in the African American population. African Americans are much more likely than their white counterparts to have diabetes. Because of the effects of diabetes and its increased prevalence in the African American population, the complication rates of diabetes are also alarmingly disproportionate. Included in these complications is stroke. Diabetes is an independent risk factor for stroke. The importance of diabetes as a risk factor in this population will continue to increase especially in areas of the United States densely populated by African Americans such as the Stroke Belt or the southeast United States. It is reasonable to conclude that stroke mortality will continue to vary by race and geographic region, with the highest variations being in the southeast African American.[9]

A second vulnerable population is the elderly. Prevention of adverse affects in the hyperglycemic elderly patient can present multiple challenges for the nurse in the intensive care unit. Adverse effects are often a result of hyperglycemic-induced immune defects and age-related immune responses.[10] Interventions must be aimed at prevention and treatment of hyperglycemia in an effort to decrease disparities in the most vulnerable populations and improve mortality rates after stroke.[11]

PATHOPHYSIOLOGIC PROCESS

The presence of type I diabetes represents a deficiency of insulin due to beta cell destruction. Type II diabetes represents a resistance to the action of insulin and an impairment of insulin secretion. Insulin plays a major role in the body's metabolism. Consequently, the absence or lack of insulin will result in hyperglycemia and have a widespread devastating effect on the body's organs and tissues. Numerous studies have indicated that brain infarct size may increase in prolonged states of hyperglycemia, and is related to increased mortality after stroke.[12]

Adequate insulin levels are strongly inhibited by norepinephrine, which subsequently leads to increased blood glucose levels during psychologic and physiologic stress. An acute stroke is a physiologic assault to the body, which causes a release of catecholamines. This release causes an increase in glycemia resulting in a natural state of hyperglycemia. This, in combination with an already poorly controlled baseline glycemia, may result in significantly elevated blood glucose levels. A prolonged state of hyperglycemia causes prolonged acidosis and failure of high-energy phosphate metabolism.[13] Ischemic brain cells already undergoing anaerobic metabolic processes are at risk for significantly worse injury when exposed to systemic acidosis caused by hyperglycemia. The eventual progression from acidosis to alkalosis has been found to correlate with a decline in neurologic function.[14]

Glycemic control plays a major role in both micro- and macrovascular disease. Often problems with microvascular circulation are thought to be caused by macrovascular problems. However, it is the damage to the small blood vessels of the body, which leads to widespread vascular damage that impedes blood flow to vital organs such as the brain. This macrovascular damage results in stroke and ultimately may lead to death (**Fig. 1**).

GLUCOSE CONTROL METHODS FOR ACUTE CARE

Formerly, strict glycemic control in acutely ill patients may have presented a venue for debate. However, the need for reasonably aggressive therapy in certain acute illnesses such as stroke has brought increased attention to management in the inpatient setting. The American Diabetes Association (ADA) 2009 guidelines support glucose levels of less than 140 mg/dL in medical intensive care units (**Table 1**). In addition, much of the current literature supports the importance of tight glycemic control in the critically ill. This focus has resulted in implementation of practice guidelines in acute care settings across the United States that aims to control strictly blood glucose levels. Recent clinical trials aimed at evaluating the effectiveness of tight glycemic control are included in (**Table 2**).

There are reliable methods available to control blood glucose levels in the acute stroke patient. However, the benefits associated with some of the more traditional methods should be questioned because of significantly limited glycemic control during physiologic stress. For example, in severe states of hyperglycemia, use of subcutaneous insulin therapy 4 times daily or as needed may result in lack of control of blood glucose. In fact, sliding-scale insulin is not recommended because it is ineffective and potentially dangerous.[21]

On the other hand, more aggressive continuous intravenous insulin therapy results in improved glycemic levels with less variability, rendering this form of treatment as much more suitable in acute stroke patients with significant hyperglycemia. Ideally, a standard algorithm for blood glucose monitoring during intravenous insulin therapy should be followed and monitored by nursing personnel. A number of protocols are available in the literature that support safe management of patients receiving continuous insulin infusions, consisting of hourly glucose monitoring to achieve safe glycemic control.

The benefits of glycemic control on morbidity reduction through implementation of intravenous insulin protocols administered using evidence-based practice algorithms

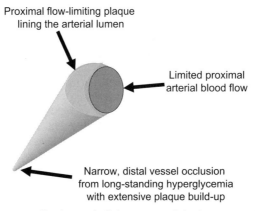

Fig. 1. Macrovascular complications of diabetes: arterial plaque associated with poorly controlled blood glucose.

| Table 1 ||| |
| ADA recommendations for glucose control in the hospital setting ||| |
2009 ADA Guidelines	**Intensive Care**	**Medical or Surgical Wards**
Known diabetics	Surgical: blood glucose levels as close to 110 mg/dL and generally <140 mg/dL Medical: blood glucose levels <140 mg/dL	Fasting glucose <126 mg/dL Random glucose >180–200 mg/dL
No known history of diabetes	Surgical: blood glucose levels as close to 10 mg/dL and generally <140 mg/dL Medical: blood glucose levels <140 mg/dL	Fasting glucose <126 mg/dL Random glucose >180–200 mg/dL

Data from American Diabetes Association, 2009.

are well described in the literature. Greater benefits have been achieved with glycemic reductions in the range of 108 mg/dL to 180 mg/dL and have yielded a reduction in mortality, yet must be balanced against the risk for hypoglycemic events when especially tight controls (reduction to below 110 mg/dL) are used. While other glycemic control methods exist that involve lifestyle modifications (eg, weight loss, stress reduction, regular exercise, and smoking cessation), cases of severe hyperglycemia are beyond use of these methods, which should be reserved for the recovery phase of stroke.

The American Heart Association (AHA) and ADA provide evidence-based recommendations for primary and secondary stroke prevention and management through glycemic control. Glucose control is recommended to near-normoglycemic levels (110–140 mg/dL) among diabetics with ischemic stroke or transient ischemic attack in an effort to prevent macrovascular complications.[22] The AHA identifies the goal for hemoglobin A1c at less than or equal to 7%.

After severe hyperglycemic states have been corrected, transition to oral agents may be considered if appropriate. Some oral agents have been shown to be very effective in glycemic control, but these agents may be inappropriate in the stroke patient with dysphagia. In addition, oral agents may result in glucose levels higher than desired in an effort to avoid hypoglycemia, and may carry significant side effects such as weight gain, intestinal upset, headache, and hypersensitivity.

Sulfonylurea agents require dosing 2 or 3 times daily, and may also be teratogenic, but the second-generation sulfonylureas have fewer side effects but are more expensive. It has been hypothesized by some researchers that patients on sulfonylureas pre- and poststroke have better outcomes,[23] and these benefits have been observed in patients with nonlacunar strokes. Other oral agents include meglitinides, biguanides, thiazolidinediones, and alpha-glucosidase inhibitors with adverse effects including hypoglycemia, lactic acidosis, edema, and gastrointestinal upset.

Long-acting insulin may also play an important role in the long-term management of hyperglycemia. Long-acting insulin given once a day closely resembles normal basal insulin produced by the pancreas. Generally, the use of long-acting insulin requires the addition of other interventions to sufficiently lower blood glucose and is insufficient as monotherapy. Premixed insulin, though effective in decreasing blood sugar, carries the unwanted risk of side effects such as weight gain.

Table 2 Glucose control clinical trials		
Research Study	**Research Design**	**Research Findings**
NICE-SUGAR trial, 2009[15]	Randomized controlled trial	Blood glucose target of less than 180 mg/dL resulted in lower mortality than a target of 81 to 108 mg/dL. Strict glycemic control below 108 increased adult mortality in the ICU.
Tight glycemic control by an automated algorithm with time-variant sampling in medical ICU patients, 2008[16]	Randomized controlled trial	Computer-based enhanced model predictive control (eMPC) algorithm was effective in maintaining tight glycemic control in severely ill medical ICU patients.
Treatment of Hyperglycemia in Ischemic Stroke (THIS), 2008[17]	Randomized controlled pilot study	The intravenous insulin protocol corrected hyperglycemia in patients with acute ischemic stroke significantly better than usual care without major adverse events.
Intensive insulin therapy in the medical ICU 2006[18]	Randomized controlled trial	Intensive insulin therapy significantly reduced morbidity, but not mortality among all patients in the medical ICU.
The Hyperglycemia: Intensive Insulin Infusion in Infarction (HI-5) study, 2006[19]	Randomized control trial	No reduction in mortality among patients who received insulin or dextrose infusion therapy.
SPRINT (Specialized Relative Insulin and Nutrition Tables) protocol, 2006[20]	Quasi-experimental pilot study, using an historical control group	SPRINT achieved a high level of glycemic control on a severely ill clinical population with a significantly lower mortality rate when compared with the historical hyperglycemic control group. Unlike historical controls, range and peak blood glucose metrics were not correlated with mortality outcome in subjects on the SPRINT protocol.

GOAL GLYCEMIC TARGET DEBATED

There is currently a debate over how tightly controlled blood glucose should be in critically ill patients. This is fueled by complications associated with glucose levels below 110 mg/dL. A recently published meta-analysis of 29 studies reviewed the benefits

Box 1
Example of a continuous intravenous insulin infusion algorithm

Target range for glycemic control: 110–140 mg/dL

Routine infusion 100 units insulin/100 mL 0.9% NaCl.

IV insulin—regular or NovoLog

Begin IV insulin infusion when blood glucose is at or above 140 mg/dL

Insulin infusions should be discontinued when

Patient is receiving <0.5 units/h

Use "noncritical care setting" algorithm for management of daily basal insulin, supplemental, and prandial insulin.

Patient should receive a bolus dose

Obtain random blood sugar. Divide random blood sugar level by 100. For values greater than 0.5 may round to nearest 1.0 unit. For values less than 0.5 round down to nearest 1.0 unit.

Example: patient's blood sugar is 275 ÷ 100 = 2.75 rounds up to 3 units.

Bolus dose = 3 units of regular or NovoLog Insulin

Initial infusion rate

Patient's initial IV infusion rate should be started at the same number of units as the bolus dose. Example: the IV infusion rate should start at 3 units/h

Intravenous fluids

Start dextrose 5% water (D5W) @ 100 cc/h

If patient receiving total parenteral nutrition (TPN) or enteral feedings do not start D5W. An equivalent rate of 10 g glucose/h is required

Glucose units per hour

350–400 4 units

300–349 3 units

270–299 3 units

250–269 3 units

230–249 2 units

210–229 2 units

190–209 2 units

150–189 2 units

110–149 1 unit

<110 OFF

Algorithm 2 for patients not controlled with Algorithm 1 or patients receiving >100 units per d of outpatient insulin

Glucose units per hour

350–400 4.5 units

300–349 3.5 units

270–299 3.5 units

250–269 3.5 units

230–249 2.5 units

210–229 2.5 units

190–209 2.5 units

150–189 2.5 units

110–149 1.5 units

<110 OFF

Algorithm 3 for patients not controlled with Algorithm 2. Must receive order from endocrinology service before initiation.

Glucose units per hour

350–400 5units

300–349 4units

270–299 4units

250–269 3 units

230–249 3 units

210–229 3 units

190–209 3 units

150–189 3 units

110–149 2 units

<110 OFF

Blood glucose monitoring

Hourly venous punctures until glucose <400 mg/dL; then finger sticks every hour until glucose is within goal x 6 h; then every 2 h x 6 h; Then every 4 h for remainder of therapy.

If any change in insulin infusion rate or significant changes in clinical condition, resume hourly glucose monitoring until glucose is again stable.

and risks of tight glucose control versus usual care in critically ill adult patients. The results revealed that extremely tight glucose control was not associated with a significant reduction in hospital mortality, but was associated with a significant increased risk of hypoglycemia.[24] The recent international randomized clinical trial, NICE-SUGAR[15] revealed somewhat similar results, with extremely tight glucose control (blood glucose 81–108 mg/dL) being associated with increased mortality in critically ill patients.

While the patient samples in these trials were not limited exclusively to stroke, it is probably sound to generalize these findings to acute diabetic stroke patients. In an effort to prevent the untoward effects of hypoglycemia, blood glucose in acute stroke should be maintained between 110 and 140 mg/dL. This range of blood sugar can be successfully maintained through diligent monitoring and treatment supported by a prudent algorithm, resulting in near normoglycemia, with decreased morbidity and mortality (**Box 1**).

SUMMARY

Primary and secondary prevention are important in glycemic control and stroke prevention. When high levels of glucose are left untreated in stroke patients, ischemic neurologic damage may be exacerbated. Maintaining reasonably consistent strict glycemic control in the acutely ill patient is crucial for optimal recovery.

Hyperglycemia, is a prevalent complication in critically ill patients, and has been shown to have a negative influence on morbidity and mortality. The use of reasonably aggressive intravenous insulin therapy does appear to improve patient outcomes in states of severe hyperglycemia, but requires cautious monitoring and management to prevent hypoglycemia. While findings from large multisite, randomized controlled trials of tight glycemic control in subjects that are exclusively acute strokes are lacking, generalization of findings from other acute care patients to the acute stroke population is rational, until data emerge that may warrant a change in this practice.

REFERENCES

1. Capes SE, Hunt D, Malmberg K, et al. Stress hyperglycemia and prognosis of stroke in nondiabetic and diabetic patients: a systemic review. Stroke 2001;32: 2426–32.
2. Wild S, Roglic G, Green A, et al. Global prevalence of diabetes. Diabetes Care 2004;27(5):1047–53.
3. American Diabetes Association Website. Diabetes statistics. Available at: http://www.diabetes.org/diabetes-statistics.jsp. Accessed July 22, 2008.
4. Kannel WB, McGee DL. Diabetes and cardiovascular disease: the Framingham Study. JAMA 1979;241(19):2035–8.
5. American Stroke Association Website. How cardiovascular and stroke risk relate. Available at: http://www.strokeassociation.org/presenter.jhtml?identifier= 3027411. Accessed July 22, 2008.
6. American Diabetes Association Website. Diabetes: heart disease and stroke. Available at: http://www.diabetes.org/diabetes-heart-disease-stroke.jsp. Accessed July 22, 2008.
7. National Diabetes International Clearinghouse. National diabetes statistics, 2007. Available at: http://diabetes.niddk.nih.gov/dm/pubs/statistics/#complications. Accessed August 1, 2008.
8. American Heart Association. Stroke statistics. Available at: http://www.american-heart.org/presenter.jhtml?identifier=4725. Accessed August 1, 2008.
9. Voeks JH, McClure LA, Go RC, et al. Regional differences in diabetes as a possible contributor to the geographic disparity in stroke mortality. Stroke 2008;39(6):1675–80.
10. Szerszen A, Castellanos MR, Seminara DP. Glucose control in the hospitalized elderly—a concern not just for patients with diabetes. Geriatrics 2009;64(6): 18–20.
11. Gentile NT, Seftchick MW. Poor outcomes in hispanic and African American patients after ischemic stroke: influence of diabetes and hyperglycemia. Ethn Dis 2008;18(3):330–5.
12. Kes VB, Solter VV, Supanc V, et al. Impact of hyperglycemia on ischemic stroke mortality in diabetic and non-diabetic patients. Ann Saudi Med 2007;27(5):352.
13. Levine SR, Welch KM, Helpern JA, et al. Prolonged deterioration of ischemic brain energy metabolism and acidosis associated with hyperglycemia: human cerebral infarction studied by serial 31P NMR spectroscopy. Ann Neurol 1988; 23(4):416–8.
14. Welch KM, Levine SR, Helpern JA. Pathophysiological correlates of cerebral ischemia the significance of cellular acid base shifts. Funct Neurol 1990;5(1): 21–31.
15. The NICE-SUGAR Study Investigators. Intensive versus conventional glucose control in critically ill patient. N Engl J Med 2009;360(13):1283–97.

16. Pachler C, Plank J, Weinhandl H, et al. Tight glycaemic control by an automated algorithm with time-variant sampling in medical ICU patients. Intensive Care Med 2008;34(7):1224–30.
17. Bruno A, Kent TA, Coull BM, et al. Treatment of hyperglycemia in ischemic stroke (THIS): a randomized pilot trial. Stroke 2008;39(2):384–9.
18. Van den Berghe G, Wilmer A, Hermans G, et al. Intensive insulin therapy in the medical ICU. N Engl J Med 2006;354(5):449–61.
19. Cheung NW, Wong VW, McLean M. The Hyperglycemia: Intensive Insulin Infusion in Infarction (HI-5) Study: a randomized controlled trial of insulin infusion therapy for myocardial infarction. Diabetes Care 2006;29(4):765–70.
20. Lonergan T, Compte AL, Willacy M, et al. A pilot study of the SPRINT protocol for tight glycemic control in critically ill patients. Diabetes Technol Ther 2006;8(4): 449–62.
21. Hassan E. Hyperglycemia management in the hospital setting. Am J Health Syst Pharm 2007;64:s9–14.
22. Sacco RL, Adams R, Albers G, et al. Guidelines for prevention of stroke in patients with ischemic stroke or transient ischemic attack. Stroke 2006;37(2): 577–617.
23. Kunte H, Schmidt S, Eliasziw M, et al. Sulfonylureas improve outcome in patients with type 2 diabetes and acute ischemic stroke. Stroke 2007;38(9):2526–30.
24. Wiener RS, Wiener DC, Larson RJ. Benefits and risks of tight glucose control in critically ill adults: a meta-analysis. JAMA 2008;300(8):933–44.

Antiplatelets and Stroke Outcomes: State of the Science

Dawn Meyer, MSN, FNP, RN, PhD(c)

KEYWORDS

- Antiplatelets • Stroke • Medications

Antiplatelet medications are currently used in the secondary prevention of ischemic stroke. These medications serve to prevent the formation of emboli and thrombus to avert further vascular occlusion and ischemia. The antiplatelet medications aspirin, clopidogrel (Plavix®), and extended release aspirin/dipyridamole (Aggrenox®) represent the mainstay of secondary prevention of ischemic stroke and transient ischemic attack (TIA). Although antiplatelet medications prevent platelet aggregation by different mechanisms, the end result is a significant decrease in the risk of secondary stroke, myocardial infarction (MI), and death.[1-3] Increasingly, the literature reflects hypotheses about the potential utility of aspirin (acetylsalicylic acid [ASA]) and clopidogrel antiplatelet therapy, as a preventative measure in patients at risk of stroke and as an approach to treat embolic ischemic stroke in the acute phase once it has occurred.[4] This article reviews the use of antiplatelets in secondary stroke prevention and in acute stroke treatment.

CURRENT ANTIPLATELET USE IN STROKE

Current evidence does not support the usefulness of antiplatelet medications as a primary prevention measure for stroke. To this end, the current approved use of antiplatelet medications in stroke is as a secondary prevention measure.[5] Current guidelines for prevention of recurrent stroke state that the use of aspirin (50–325 mg/d) monotherapy, aspirin and extended-release dipyridamole in combination (Aggrenox), or clopidogrel (Plavix) monotherapy are all acceptable options for initial therapy.[5]

Aspirin (50–1300 mg/day) has been shown to be effective as a secondary prevention measure in multiple randomized clinical trials.[2,6] The combination of extended release dipyridamole and aspirin (Aggrenox) has been shown to reduce the risk of stroke and death by 33% and the risk of stroke alone by 38%, as compared with placebo. A subsequent trial of extended release dipyridamole and aspirin (Aggrenox) versus aspirin alone showed a risk reduction of 18% with aspirin alone and 37% with

Sharp Memorial Hospital, Ortho/Neuro Services, 7901 Frost Street, San Diego, CA 92123, USA
E-mail address: dawn.matherne@sharp.com

Crit Care Nurs Clin N Am 21 (2009) 517–528
doi:10.1016/j.ccell.2009.07.016   ccnursing.theclinics.com
0899-5885/09/$ – see front matter © 2009 Elsevier Inc. All rights reserved.

Aggrenox.[2] When compared with aspirin, clopidogrel has been shown to be safe and decrease the risk of a composite outcome of ischemic stroke, MI, or vascular death by 8.7% ($P = .043$).[1] Although aspirin has been shown to be inferior when compared with Aggrenox and Plavix, its use is still recommended given its relative effectiveness and superior cost profile when compared with other medications.[7] Based on 2 large randomized controlled trials, the long-term use of aspirin and clopidogrel in combination is not recommended as a means of secondary stroke prevention, because the combination showed no superiority in preventing ischemic events and showed a twofold increase in bleeding events.[8,9] Of most concern was a significant increase (absolute risk increase 1.3%) in symptomatic intracranial hemorrhage (sICH), defined as the presence of bleeding within the brain tissue accompanied by a clinical neurologic worsening. Although long-term use of aspirin plus clopidogrel has been shown to significantly increase bleeding risk, acute, short-term use of aspirin and clopidogrel as a treatment measure, particularly in loading doses, has not been fully examined in the acute stroke population.

Thus, the efficacy of antiplatelet medications for secondary prevention of stroke has been well described in the literature. Yet few studies have assessed their use as an acute therapy for ischemic stroke.[4,10] The effectiveness of these agents is based on their pharmacologic activity in hemostasis and thrombus formation; thus, the mechanism of action of the medications, ASA and clopidogrel, is first considered.

Aspirin

Synthetic ASA, marketed as aspirin, has antipyretic, analgesic, anti-inflammatory, and antiplatelet properties. The antiplatelet effects of aspirin were first described by Gibson[11] and Craven,[12] who reported protective benefits with respect to stroke and MI. Because of its usefulness as an antiplatelet medication and its cost of approximately $0.01 per 81 to 325 mg dose, aspirin has become a cornerstone of secondary prevention in ischemic stroke and TIA.[13,14]

Antiplatelet mechanism of action of aspirin

The overall mechanism of the antiplatelet action of aspirin involves its blocking of arachidonic acid production, thereby halting thromboxane A_2 and prostaglandin biosynthesis in clot formation (**Fig. 1**).[15] Thromboxane A_2 and prostaglandin production are mediated by 2 key enzymes, cyclooxygenase-1 and -2 (COX-1 and COX 2). COX-1 is an enzyme that is present in most mammalian cells and is responsible for the production of prostanoids, such as prostaglandin, thromboxane, and prostacyclin. COX-2 is induced in response to inflammation and also produces the prostanoid molecules (PI_2-PF_2).

Both COX enzymes convert arachidonic acid to prostaglandin H_2 (PGH_2), the precursor of the prostanoids. As seen in **Fig. 1**, the metabolism of arachidonic acid by the PGH pathways results in the expression of multiple prostaglandins (PGI_2, PGE_2, PGD_2, and $PGF_{2\alpha}$) and thromboxane A_2.[16] Aspirin inhibits COX-1 and COX-2 and therefore inhibits the products of their activation, thromboxane A and prostaglandin. The thromboxane pathway induced by arachidonic acid is primary to platelet activation (see **Fig. 1**).

Aspirin's inhibitory effect on prostaglandin synthesis, and therefore platelet activation, results primarily from its inhibition of the COX enzymes (**Fig. 2**). These enzymes are physiologically active for responses other than arachidonic acid degradation, which may be adversely affected with the administration of aspirin. COX-1 is constitutional and involved in the regulation of renal blood flow and protection of gastric mucosa, platelet activation, and platelet aggregation through platelet surface receptor

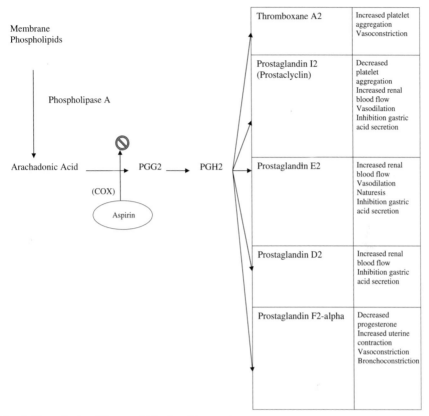

Fig. 1. The effects of the arachidonic acid cascade.

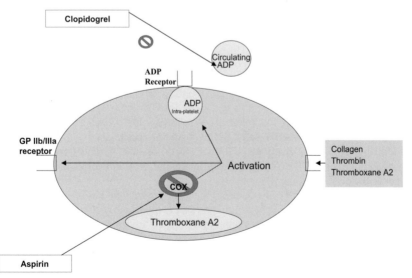

Fig. 2. Sites of action of the antiplatelet medications aspirin and clopidogrel on platelet surface receptors.

activation. COX-2 is induced by growth factors and cytokines and results in the synthesis of prostaglandins that mediate the inflammatory response.[17] When aspirin is administered, neither COX-1 nor COX-2 can degrade arachidonic acid. Although aspirin permanently inhibits COX-1 and COX-2, its inhibition of COX-1 is 170 times greater than that of COX-2.[18] Thus, inhibition of COX-1 accounts for the antiplatelet mechanism of action of aspirin, whereas inhibition of COX-2 accounts for its anti-inflammatory effects.[19]

Although the use of aspirin as a secondary stroke prevention medication is based on its inhibition of thromboxane A_2 and prostaglandin production, other mechanisms have been suggested that may account for the clinical benefit of aspirin in patients at risk of stroke and other vascular occlusive diseases. Some studies have shown that aspirin may also mildly inhibit atherosclerotic plaque generation, by making low density lipo-proteins less likely to oxidize and be taken up by macrophages to form atherosclerotic plaques.[20] Some evidence supports the role of COX-2 in protection against atheroscle-rotic plaque rupture in animal models of stroke; however, its main role is in inflammatory response rather than platelet activation.[21] The inhibition of prostaglandin synthesis by aspirin has also been found to increase nitric oxide production through the activation of neutrophils, which results in vasodilatation and increased perfusion.[22]

Limitations of aspirin as a monotherapeutic antiplatelet medication

Despite the low cost and demonstrated benefit of aspirin in secondary prevention of clot formation, there are significant limitations to its use. Specifically, aspirin is an incomplete platelet inhibitor in that it only blocks thromboxane-dependent platelet activation and aggregation; other coagulation processes can still occur in the absence of thromboxane. For example, platelet activation can be precipitated by increased pressure and shear force in the vessel wall or by increased plasma levels of catechol-amines, thrombin, and adenosine diphosphate (ADP); platelets can continue to be activated even when aspirin levels peak.[23] Furthermore, aspirin-induced inhibition of COX-2 may also increase the risks associated with atherosclerosis. COX-2 provides protection from atherosclerotic plaque rupture in murine models, which may explain the increased risk of stroke, MI, and death seen in patients taking selective COX-2 inhibitors.[21]

Clopidogrel (Plavix)

Antiplatelet mechanism of action of clopidogrel

Clopidogrel belongs to the family of antiplatelet medications called thienopyridines, which also includes ticlopidine (Ticlid®). Thienopyridines prevent platelet aggregation and clot formation by acting as antagonists at the P2 receptor located on the platelet surface, thereby blocking the release of ADP (**Fig. 3**).[24] Although a weak platelet agonist in itself, ADP that is secreted by platelets amplifies the platelet response induced by other platelet agonists such as thromboxane A_2 and thrombin. It is the amplifying effect of ADP on platelet aggregation that accounts for its key role in hemo-stasis and clot formation.[25]

Of the P2 receptor subtypes, $P2Y_{12}$ has been identified as having a key role in thrombus formation.[26] The activation of the $P2Y_{12}$ receptor by circulating ADP causes a release of intraplatelet ADP, resulting in a positive feedback loop (see **Fig. 3**). Acti-vation of this receptor by intraplatelet ADP leads to platelet aggregation, and it is this receptor subtype that is antagonized by clopidogrel.

Thus, the overall mechanism of action by which clopidogrel inhibits ADP-induced platelet aggregation is by blocking the P_2Y_{12} receptor release of ADP (see **Fig. 3**). This antagonism results in 3 distinct methods of inhibiting platelet aggregation. First,

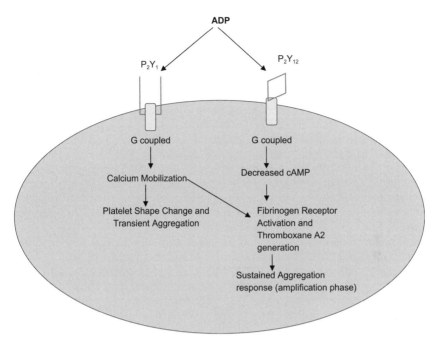

Fig. 3. The effects of ADP platelet surface receptor activation.

this blockade does not allow for the platelet shape change needed for platelet aggregation and clot formation. Second, the release of ADP fails to be amplified. Finally, the platelet-aggregating effects of thromboxane A_2, thrombin, and other platelet agonists are diminished by inhibiting ADP's magnification of their effects.[27–29]

Limitations of clopidogrel as a monotherapeutic antiplatelet medication

The major limitations of clopidogrel as an antiplatelet medication relate to its specific G protein-coupled pathway platelet inhibition, its specific ADP receptor blockade, and its cost. Clopidogrel specifically inhibits the G pathway. This is a specific method of receptor activation, whereby the ligand is transported to the cell nucleus to effect transcriptional change. Multitudes of cell receptors that are vital to life processes are activated in the G pathway; therefore, a complete blockade of this pathway is lethal.

As is the case with aspirin, clopidogrel alone does not offer complete platelet inhibition because platelets can be activated by multiple surface receptors (see **Fig. 2**). Despite these multiple paths, activation of the glycoprotein IIb/IIIa complex (GPIIb-IIIa) receptor is the final common step in platelet aggregation (see **Fig. 2**).[30] The use of GPIIb-IIIa inhibitors as a method of antiplatelet therapy will be discussed later in this article; however, the combined use of 2 antiplatelets with different mechanisms of action, such as aspirin and clopidogrel, serves to prevent the ultimate activation of the GPIIb-IIIa receptor and to prevent platelet aggregation. The use of clopidogrel alone does not provide blockade of the final common pathway of platelet activation.

The cost of clopidogrel has also been discussed as a limitation of its use as an antiplatelet therapy. When compared with the per dose cost of aspirin ($0.02), clopidogrel is significantly costlier at approximately $2.50 per dose.[13] Studies such as clopidogrel versus aspirin in patients at risk of ischemic events (CAPRIE) have demonstrated the statistically significant health benefits of clopidogrel therapy when compared with aspirin,[1] but its cost-effectiveness is less clear. Although most studies have reported that clopidogrel use is not cost-effective in secondary stroke prevention, 2 studies have shown a cost benefit in high-risk acute coronary syndrome patients.[31,32]

Extended Release Dipyridamole Plus Aspirin (Aggrenox)

Antiplatelet mechanism of action of extended release dipyridamole plus aspirin (Aggrenox)

Aggrenox, which contains 200 mg extended release dipyridamole and 25 mg aspirin, belongs to the family of pyrimidopyrimidine derivatives. The mechanism of action is through vasodilatory and antiplatelet properties. The proposed pathways of action include inhibition of phosphodiesterase, which increases cyclic guanosine monophosphate (cGMP), and blocking of adenosine uptake into the cell, which increases intraplatelet cyclic adenosine monophosphate (cAMP), resulting in platelet inhibition.

Three major studies have supported the use of Aggrenox as a means of secondary stroke prevention. The European Stroke Prevention Study (ESPS)-2 enrolled 6602 subjects with prior stroke or TIA. The 4 treatment groups included placebo, aspirin 25 mg bid, extended release dipyridamole 200 mg bid, and a combination of extended release dipyridamole (200 mg) and aspirin (25 mg). Relative risk reduction over placebo was 18% for low dose aspirin ($P = .013$), 16.3% for extended release dipyridamole alone ($P = .039$), and 37% with the combination of extended release dipyridamole and aspirin ($P<.001$). The number needed to treat with Aggrenox to prevent 1 stroke is 18 when compared to placebo and 34 compared with aspirin alone.

The European-Australian Stroke Prevention in Reversible Ischemia Trials (ESPRIT and ESPRIT-2) assessed the efficacy of Aggrenox versus aspirin in the prevention of death from all vascular causes, nonfatal stroke, nonfatal MI, or major bleeding complication. Subjects were randomized to receive either Aggrenox bid (n = 1363) or daily aspirin (n = 1376). The primary outcome occurred in 13% (n = 173) of the Aggrenox group and in 16% of the aspirin-alone group. The use of Aggrenox led to a hazard ratio (HR) of 0.80 compared with the use of aspirin alone and an absolute risk reduction of 1% per year. When compared with oral anticoagulation therapy (international normalized ratio [INR] 2-3), a 24% relative risk reduction was seen in the Aggrenox group. This provided evidence that the use of Aggrenox in this population was superior to treatment with anticoagulation.

Finally, the Prevention Regimen for Successfully Avoiding Second Strokes (PRoFESS) study compared the relative efficacy and safety of aspirin plus extended-release dipyridamole (Aggrenox) to clopidogrel among patients who had suffered a recent ischemic stroke, for the primary outcome of recurrent stroke. Over 5 years, 20,332 patients were randomized to Aggrenox bid (n = 10,181) or clopidogrel daily (n = 10,151). The total number of recurrent strokes was 1814: Aggrenox 9% (n = 916) and clopidogrel 8.8% (n = 898) (HR, 1.01; confidence interval [CI], 0.92–1.11). Because the CI extended beyond 1.075, the prespecified noninferiority endpoint was not met. Medication compliance was 69.6% in the Aggrenox group versus 76.8% in the clopidogrel group. A per protocol analysis revealed recurrence rates of 7.6% with Aggrenox and 7.7% with clopidogrel, which were not statistically significant. There was no significant difference in 3-month modified Rankin scale (mRS) grades of 3 or higher between the groups (4.1% Aggrenox, 3.9% clopidogrel); mRS is an ordinal functional outcome scale, which is used in most stroke trials. Major hemorrhagic events occurred more frequently among Aggrenox but there was no significant difference between groups (4.1% Aggrenox vs 3.6% clopidogrel; HR, 1.15; 95% CI, 1.00–1.32). Examining all intracranial hemorrhage (ICH) showed significantly greater frequency in patients receiving Aggrenox (1.4% Aggrenox vs 1.0% clopidogrel; HR, 1.42; 95% CI, 1.11–1.83; P = .006).

EFFICACY OF ACUTE ANTIPLATELET LOADING

Although aspirin and clopidogrel have limitations when used as monotherapy for secondary stroke prevention, the acute use of these medications together in large doses may prove effective in acute stroke treatment as opposed to stroke prevention. As previously reviewed, the efficacy of the antiplatelet medications aspirin and clopidogrel for secondary prevention of stroke has been well described; preliminary evidence of their safety and efficacy in the acute treatment of stroke has emerged.[4,10] Proposed evaluation of these antiplatelet agents as an acute therapy for ischemic stroke is based on (1) evidence for antiplatelet loading efficacy in the acute treatment of vascular occlusive coronary disease; (2) the acute efficacy of other intravenous antiplatelet medications, abciximab and heparin, for the treatment of ischemic stroke; and (3) preliminary evidence for the efficacy of aspirin and clopidogrel loading in acute ischemic stroke and transient ischemic attack.

Use of Antiplatelet Loading in the Ischemic Stroke Population

Extrapolation from the cardiology literature has resulted in evaluation of acute antiplatelet therapy for ischemic stroke patients. Several clinical trials have assessed the safety of acute antiplatelet medications other than ASA and clopidogrel in ischemic stroke. The initial study of acute antiplatelet treatment in ischemic stroke involved the use of GPIIb-IIIa inhibitors. As the final common step of platelet activation (see **Fig. 2**), these medications seemed a logical choice as an effective therapy. The Abciximab in Acute Ischemic Stroke trial (AbESTT) was a randomized, double-blind, placebo-controlled Phase IIb trial of abciximab (ReoPro) in 400 adult patients with acute ischemic stroke who were able to be treated within 6 hours of stroke onset (Abciximab Emergent Stroke treatment Trial AbESTT Investigators, 2005). The co-primary endpoints of the trial were fatal or symptomatic ICH rates at day 5 or at discharge (whichever was sooner) and the clinical outcome at 3 months as measured on the mRS, with scores of 0 to 6 (where 0 is normal and 6 is death). The National Institutes of Health Stroke Scale (NIHSS), an ordinal scale of stroke severity with scores of 0 for normal and 42 for highest stroke severity, was also used to classify patients by stroke severity. Analysis of mRS responders was a prespecified secondary analysis, with "responders" defined as (1) mRS at 3 months = 0, if NIHSS score at baseline was 4 to 7; (2) mRS at 3 months = 0 to 1, if NIHSS score at baseline was 8 to 14; and (3) mRS at 3 months = 0, 1, or 2, if NIHSS score at baseline was 15 to 22. Researchers found no sICH within 5 days after treatment; asymptomatic hemorrhages occurred at rates of 7% in the treatment group versus 5% in the placebo group (P>.05). Significantly more patients treated with abciximab within 5 hours of the onset of stroke achieved mRS scores of 0 or 1 (normal or near-normal function) than placebo (53.9% vs 34.6%; P = .013).A post hoc analysis revealed that patients treated with abciximab within a 5-hour window had a larger therapeutic benefit as compared with patients treated more than 5 hours after symptom onset; 53.9% of patients treated within 5 hours with abciximab achieved mRS of 0 or 1 at 3 months versus 34.6% treated with placebo (odds ratio [OR], 2.21; 95% CI, 1.18–4; P = .013). If treatment was started after 5 hours, 43.4% of abciximab-treated patients and 44.1% of placebo-treated patients achieved mRS of 0 or 1 at 3 months (OR, 1.03; 95% CI, 0.61–1.73; P>.05).

The subsequent AbESTT II trial was a phase III, randomized, double-blind comparison of abciximab versus placebo given as a bolus (0.25 mg/kg), followed by a 12-hour infusion (0.125 µg/kg/min, 10 µg/min maximum), in patients presenting within 5 or 6 hours of stroke onset. The trial also included a third group of patients who awoke with stroke symptoms and could be randomized within 2.5 hours. The trial was halted in May 2005 because of an increased risk of sICH. At 3 months, approximately 33% of patients assigned placebo (72/218) and 32% of patients assigned abciximab (71/221; P = .944) in the primary cohort were judged to have a favorable response to treatment. The distributions of outcomes on the mRS were similar between the treated and control groups. Within 5 days of enrollment, approximately 5.5% of abciximab-treated and 0.5% of placebo-treated patients in the primary cohort had symptomatic or fatal ICH (P = .002). The trial also failed to demonstrate an improvement in outcomes with abciximab among patients in the companion and wake-up cohorts. Although the number of patients was small, an increased rate of hemorrhage was noted within 5 days among patients in the wake-up population who received abciximab (13.6% vs 5% for placebo). The trial had been in the enrollment phase at 150 international sites since 2003, with a target enrollment of 1800 patients. Expert review of the results revealed that the most likely cause of ICH was the high dose of abciximab used in the trial.[33]

In a later trial, Mandava and colleagues[34] studied the safety of abciximab and heparin infusion for patients within 6 hours of anterior circulation symptoms and 24 hours of basilar artery thrombosis. Researchers enrolled 14 patients with ischemic stroke, ineligible for intravenous (IV) recombinant tissue plasminogen activator (rt-PA). An initial IV bolus of 0.20 mg/kg of abciximab was given over 1 minute. Subsequently, the treatment team decided on whether to administer an IV infusion of abciximab over 12 hours at a dose of 0.05 µg/kg/min, along with weight-adjusted heparin; the decision was based on clinical judgment regarding ongoing hemorrhage risks. The dose was chosen based on results from the initial phase II trial with abciximab, which showed fewer asymptomatic hemorrhages and only marginal difference in outcome compared with higher doses. Mean age of the subjects was 57 (range, 39–82), with 9 men and 5 women. Mean NIHSS score before treatment was 22, median 22 (range, 7–37). Mean time to treat from onset was 4.4 hours (range, 2.15–13). Researchers found no symptomatic hemorrhages and one asymptomatic basal ganglia hemorrhage, which was discovered by routine computed tomographic scan 31 hours after abciximab treatment. Mean improvement in NIHSS score was 10.7 (range, 0–22). A larger safety and efficacy trial has not been performed on this regimen; therefore, it is not used in clinical practice.

The study of intravenous acute antiplatelet therapy has not translated into a change in clinical practice due to lack of efficacy and safety concerns. The lack of benefit seen with intravenous GPIIb-IIIa antagonists and heparins may be due to either dosing or improper receptor targeting (see **Fig. 2**). The dosing used in the AbESTT trial was higher than that used in cardiac patients undergoing approved percutaneous coronary intervention treatments, and it may have contributed to the increased rates of bleeding seen in the phase III trial. In addition, targeting one receptor (GPIIb-IIIa) may be less beneficial than targeting multiple receptors (ie, $P2Y_{12}$, thromboxane A), given that the activation of platelets in ischemic stroke is not a single process but is more likely to occur in waves of activation and aggregation.[35]

Acute oral antiplatelet loading in ischemic stroke has been assessed in 3 clinical trials. First, the Clopidogrel and Aspirin for Reduction of Emboli in Symptomatic Carotid Stenosis (CaRESS) trial assessed clopidogrel loading (300 mg) in patients with symptomatic 50% or higher carotid stenosis, from microembolic signals (MES) on transcranial Doppler (TCD) imaging.[36] In this randomized, double-blind study, subjects were screened with TCD, and if MES was detected, they were randomized to either aspirin 75 mg or clopidogrel 300 mg and ASA 75 mg. Repeated TCD recordings were made on days 2 and 7. MES was detected in 110 of 230 patients by online analysis at baseline, of whom 107 were randomized. Analysis revealed a significant reduction in the primary end point (43.8% of dual-therapy patients were MES positive on day 7), as compared with 72.7% of monotherapy patients (relative risk reduction, 39.8%; 95% CI, 13.8–58.0; P = .0046). The secondary end point of MES frequency per hour was reduced by 61.4% (95% CI, 31.6 to 78.2; P = .0013) compared with baseline in the dual-therapy group at day 7 and by 61.6% (95% CI, 34.9–77.4; P = .0005) on day 2. There were 4 recurrent strokes and 7 TIAs in the monotherapy group versus no stroke and 4 TIAs in the dual-therapy group that was treatment-emergent and ipsilateral to the qualifying carotid stenosis; 2 additional ipsilateral TIAs occurred before treatment started. MES frequency was greater in the 17 patients with recurrent ipsilateral events compared with the 90 without (mean ± standard deviation, 24.4 ± 27.7 vs 8.9 ± 11.5 per hour; P = .0003). Although there was a significant reduction in the number of MES in the clopidogrel loading group, there were no clinical endpoints included in the trial and clinical efficacy is unknown.

The Fast Assessment of Stroke and Transient Ischemic Attack to Prevent Early Recurrence (FASTER) trial assessed whether the administration of aspirin (162 mg) and a loading dose (300 mg) followed by maintenance doses (75 mg) of clopidogrel with or without simvastatin (40 mg), within 24 hours of stroke symptom onset, reduces the risk of stroke after TIA or minor stroke (NIHSS score ≤3) at 90 days.[10] A total of 396 patients received aspirin and were then randomized in a 2 × 2 factorial design to placebo or 300 mg clopidogrel loading dose, immediately followed by 75 mg clopidogrel daily; and to placebo or 40 mg simvastatin, immediately followed by 40 mg daily. Prior use of statin was a key exclusion criterion in the study. Although the study ended early because of poor enrollment related to high rates of prior statin use, analysis of the enrolled patients revealed no significant difference in the primary outcome of stroke event rate at 90 days or in the secondary outcomes of vascular event or death at 90 days.

In a preliminary study, entitled "LOAD: A Pilot Study of the Safety of Loading of Aspirin and Clopidogrel in Acute Ischemic Stroke and TIA," Meyer and colleagues[4] examined the feasibility and safety of antiplatelet loading in acute ischemic stroke and TIA patients. Forty patients with stroke or TIA symptoms, who were not eligible for revascularization, received 375 mg clopidogrel and 325 mg aspirin within 36 hours of onset. All patients were admitted to a comprehensive stroke unit and monitored for neurologic deterioration (≥2 point increase on NIHSS score) and bleeding complications until hospital day 7 or discharge. NIHSS was performed at 24 hours postadmission and on hospital day 7 or discharge, whichever came first.

The mean time to antiplatelet loading from stroke symptom onset was 2 hours 32 minutes. Mean admission NIHSS score was 6. There were no cases of systemic hemorrhage or mortality. A single symptomatic hemorrhagic infarction (HI)-2 (2.5%) was detected 43 hours post-treatment. When compared with matched controls, loaded patients were no more likely to experience hemorrhage and significantly less likely to experience neurologic deterioration (OR, 17.2; P<.002). In this pilot trial, loading with 375 mg clopidogrel and 325 mg aspirin showed safety when administered up to 36 hours after stroke and TIA onset. Neurologic deterioration may be decreased in patients who are treated with antiplatelet loading. A need exists to examine the potential benefits of this treatment in acute cerebral ischemia.

SUMMARY

An understanding of the mechanisms of action of antiplatelet medications gives the bedside practitioner a clear rationale for the use of these medications in the secondary prevention of stroke. Despite their overall clinical benefit, one must recognize the limitations of these medications in preventing all recurrent vascular events such as stroke and MI. The evidence based care of ischemic stroke and TIA patients should include the use of aspirin (50–325 mg/d) monotherapy, aspirin and extended-release dipyridamole in combination (Aggrenox), or clopidogrel (Plavix) monotherapy as a cornerstone of an overall risk factor reduction plan. The use of oral antiplatelet loading in the ischemic stroke population has shown benefit in patients with carotid stenosis and ischemic stroke and in TIA patients who are treated within 24 hours of stroke symptom onset. The optimal time and dose of antiplatelet loading remains untested. The use of antiplatelet loading in stroke has been largely based on its success in the interventional and non-interventional cardiac population. Studies focusing on dosing, time of administration, and efficacy in ischemic stroke are needed to provide evidence for its global use in the ischemic stroke population.

REFERENCES

1. A randomised, blinded, trial of clopidogrel versus aspirin in patients at risk of ischaemic events (CAPRIE). CAPRIE Steering Committee. Lancet 1996; 348(9038):1329–39.
2. Diener HC, Cunha L, Forbes C, et al. European Stroke Prevention Study 2. Dipyridamole and acetylsalicylic acid in the secondary prevention of stroke. J Neurol Sci 1996;143:1–13.
3. The International Stroke Trial (IST): a randomised trial of aspirin, subcutaneous heparin, both, or neither among 19435 patients with acute ischaemic stroke. International Stroke Trial Collaborative Group. Lancet 1997;349:1569–81.
4. Meyer DM, Albright KC, Allison TA, et al. LOAD: a pilot study of the safety of loading of aspirin and clopidogrel in acute ischemic stroke and transient ischemic attack. J Stroke Cerebrovasc Dis 2008;17(1):26–9.
5. Adams RJ, Albers G, Alberts MJ, et al. Update to the AHA/ASA recommendations for the prevention of stroke in patients with stroke and transient ischemic attack. Stroke 2008;39(5):1647–52.
6. Collaborative overview of randomised trials of antiplatelet therapy-I: prevention of death, myocardial infarction, and stroke by prolonged antiplatelet therapy in various categories of patients. Br Med J 1994;308:81–106.
7. Sarasin FP, Gaspoz J-M, Bounameaux H. Cost-effectiveness of new antiplatelet regimens used as secondary prevention of stroke or transient ischemic attack. Arch Intern Med 2000;160(18):2773–8.
8. Diener H-C, Bogousslavsky J, Brass LM, et al. Aspirin and clopidogrel compared with clopidogrel alone after recent ischaemic stroke or transient ischaemic attack in high-risk patients (MATCH): randomised, double-blind, placebo-controlled trial. Lancet 2004;364:331–7.
9. Bhatt DL, Fox KAA, Hacke W, et al. Clopidogrel and aspirin versus aspirin alone for the prevention of atherothrombotic events. N Engl J Med 2006;354(16): 1706–17.
10. Kennedy J, Hill MD, Ryckborst KJ, et al. Fast assessment of stroke and transient ischaemic attack to prevent early recurrence (FASTER): a randomised controlled pilot trial. Lancet Neurol 2007;6(11):961–9.
11. Gibson PC. Aspirin in the treatment of vascular disease. Lancet 1949;2:1172–4.

12. Craven LL. Acetylsalicylic acid, possible prevention of coronary thrombosis. Annals of Western Medical Surgical 1950;4:95–9.

13. Schleinitz MD, Heidenreich PA. A cost-effectiveness analysis of combination anti-platelet therapy for high-risk acute coronary syndromes: clopidogrel plus aspirin versus aspirin alone. Ann Intern Med 2005;142(4):251–9.

14. Adams H, Adams R, Del Zoppo G, et al. Guidelines for the early management of patients with ischemic stroke: 2005 guidelines update a scientific statement from the Stroke Council of the American Heart Association/American Stroke Association. Stroke 2005;36(4):916–23.

15. Antman EM, DeMets D, Loscalzo J. Cyclooxygenase inhibition and cardiovascular risk. Circulation 2005;112(5):759–70.

16. Smith WL. Prostanoid biosynthesis and the mechanism of action. Am J Physiol 1992;263:F181–91.

17. Morita I, Schindler M, Regier MK, et al. Different intracellular locations for prostaglandin endoperoxide h synthase-1 and -2. J Biol Chem 1995;270(18):10902–8.

18. Vane JR, Bakhle YS, Botting RM. Cyclooxygenases 1 and 2. Annu Rev Pharmacol Toxicol 1998;38:97–120.

19. Vane JR, Botting RM. Anti-inflammatory drugs and their mechanism of action. Inflamm Res 1998;47(Suppl 2):S78–87.

20. Steer KA, Wallace TM, Bolton CH, et al. Aspirin protects low density lipoprotein from oxidative modification. Heart 1997;77(4):333–7.

21. Egan KM, Lawson JA, Fries S, et al. COX-2-derived prostacyclin confers atheroprotection on female mice. Science 2004;306(5703):1954–7.

22. Lopez-Farre A, Caramelo C, Esteban A, et al. Effects of aspirin on platelet-neutrophil interactions. Role of nitric oxide and endothelin-1. Circulation 1995;91:2080–8.

23. Folts JD, Schafer AI, Loscalzo J, et al. A perspective on the potential problems with aspirin as an antithrombotic agent: a comparison of studies in an animal model with clinical trials. J Am Coll Cardiol 1999;33(2):295–303.

24. Gachet CMD, Hechler BPD. The platelet p2 receptors in thrombosis. Semin Thromb Hemost 2005;2:162–7.

25. Ralevic V, Burnstock G. Receptors for purines and pyrimidines. Pharmacol Rev 1998;50:413–92.

26. Cattaneo M, Savage B, Ruggeri ZM. Effects of pharmacologic inhibition of P2Y1 and P2Y12 ADP receptors on shear induced platelet aggregation and platelet thrombus formation on a collagen coated surface under flow conditions. Blood 2001;98:239a.

27. Weber AA, Reimann S, Schror K. Specific inhibition of ADP-induced platelet aggregation by clopidogrel in vivo. Br J Pharmacol 1999;126:156–7.

28. Savi P, Labouret C, Delesque N, et al. $P2Y_{12}$, a new platelet ADP receptor, target of clopidogrel. Biochem Biophys Res Commun 2001;283(2):379.

29. Ferguson JJ. The role of oral antiplatelet agents in atherothrombotic disease. Am J Cardiovasc Drugs 2006;6(3):149–57.

30. Prevost N, Shattil S. Outside-in signaling by integrin alpha IIb beta 3. In: Michaels AD, editor. Platelets. 2nd edition. San Diego: Elsevier; 2007. p. 347–57.

31. Durand-Zaleski I, Bertrand ME. The value of clopidogrel versus aspirin in reducing atherthrombotic events: the CAPRIE Study. Pharmaco Economics 2004;22:19–27.

32. Karnon J, Brennon A, Pandor A, et al. Modeling the long term cost effectiveness of clopidogrel for the secondary prevention of occlusive vascular event in the UK. Curr Med Res Opin 2005;21:101–12.

33. Mandava P, Thiagarajan P, Kent TA. Glycoprotein IIb/IIIa antagonists in acute ischaemic stroke: current status and future directions. Drugs 2008;68(8):1019–28.
34. Mandava P, Lick SD, Rahman MA, et al. Initial safety experience of abciximab and heparin for acute ischemic stroke. Cerebrovasc Dis 2005;19(4):276–8.
35. Serebruany VL, Malinin AI, Oshrine BR, et al. Lack of uniform platelet activation in patients after ischemic stroke and choice of antiplatelet therapy. Thromb Res 2004;113(3–4):197–204.
36. Markus HS, Droste DW, Kaps M, et al. Dual antiplatelet therapy with clopidogrel and aspirin in symptomatic carotid stenosis evaluated using doppler embolic signal detection: the Clopidogrel and Aspirin for Reduction of Emboli in Symptomatic Carotid Stenosis (CARESS) Trial. Circulation 2005;111(17): 2233–40.

Current and Evolving Management of Subarachnoid Hemorrhage

Tracey Anderson, MSN, CNRN, FNP-BC[a,b],*

KEYWORDS

- Subarachnoid • Aneurysm • Management • Vasospasm
- Stroke

Subarachnoid hemorrhage (SAH) is a catastrophic event that carries a mortality rate of 25% to 50%,[1] with 10% to 15% of patients dying before reaching a hospital.[2] Approximately 30,000 aneurysms rupture each year in the United States.[3] Aneurysmal SAH accounts for 2% to 5% of all new strokes each year.[4] Unlike other types of strokes, the incidence of SAH has not declined over time.[5] As many as 46% of SAH survivors have long-term cognitive impairment, with impact on functional status and quality of life.[4] Modern therapy offers the opportunity to reduce the morbidity of SAH by reducing secondary injury, preventing complications, and reducing the risk of future bleeding events. For most people, an aneurysmal rupture is a life-changing event.

CAUSES OF SAH

Intracranial aneurysms are fairly common, occurring in approximately 4% of the population.[1] The incidence of SAH increases with age (mean age of approximately 50 years) and is higher in women than in men.[5] The risk of rupture depends on the size and location of the aneurysm. Smaller aneurysms (<7 mm) carry little risk in the anterior circulation, and larger aneurysms, particularly those in the posterior cerebral circulation, carry a much higher risk.[4]

SAH is classified as aneurysmal or traumatic. Ruptured aneurysm is the cause of spontaneous SAH in 85% of cases.[2] Of the remaining cases, half are attributed to nonaneurysmal perimesencephalic hemorrhage, in which blood tends to be confined to the basal cisterns and may be the result of venous bleeding or intramural dissection. The rest are due to other disorders of the blood vessels, such as arteriovenous

[a] University of Colorado Hospital, 12605 East 16th Avenue, Aurora, CO 80045, USA
[b] Department of Neurosurgery, MC 307, Academic Office Building, 12631 East 17th Avenue, Aurora, CO 80045, USA
* Department of Neurosurgery, MC 307, Academic Office Building, 12631 East 17th Avenue, Aurora, CO 80045.
E-mail address: tracey.anderson@ucdenver.edu

Crit Care Nurs Clin N Am 21 (2009) 529–539
doi:10.1016/j.ccell.2009.07.018   ccnursing.theclinics.com
0899-5885/09/$ – see front matter © 2009 Elsevier Inc. All rights reserved.

malformations, disorders of the blood vessels in the spinal cord, and bleeding into brain tumors.[2] Cocaine abuse, sickle-cell anemia, and anticoagulation use are also documented as causing SAH in some circumstances.[6]

In traumatic brain injury (TBI), it is estimated that 60% of patients have associated SAH.[2,7] TBI is linked to poorer prognosis in the setting of SAH.[7] Complications of SAH in the setting of TBI are similar to those of SAH secondary to aneurysmal rupture.

PATHOPHYSIOLOGY

Cerebral aneurysms are areas of weakness of the blood vessel wall, which often occur at a bifurcation or branch point. They are classified into the following categories: berry (saccular), inflammatory, traumatic, dissecting, neoplastic, miliary, fusiform, and those associated with arteriovenous malformations (AVMs).

Saccular aneurysms are often called "berry aneurysms," because they appear to have a neck or stem attaching them to the blood vessel. Evidence suggests that hemodynamic factors and degenerative histologic changes in the parent vessel wall contribute to aneurysm formation.[8]

Inflammatory aneurysms are either bacterial or fungal in origin, more typically occurring on distal cerebral vessels.[9] These aneurysms occur when a septic embolus lodges in a small pial vessel and initiates arteritis, followed by thrombosis, bacterial multiplication, invasion of the vessel wall, and destruction of the internal elastic lamina and media.[8]

Traumatic aneurysms occur after various types of head injury. Common locations for this type of aneurysm are the pericallosal branch of the anterior cerebral artery, the posterior cerebral artery, and the middle cerebral artery. Rupture of this type of aneurysm is associated with a 50% mortality.[8]

Dissecting aneurysms happen when a tear occurs in the intima through the media, allowing blood to collect in the subadventitial space. Occasionally, compression of the parent vessel will result in ischemia and infarction. This occurs most frequently in the middle cerebral artery and vertebral artery.[10]

Neoplastic aneurysms result from tumor invasion of the vessel wall followed by tumor embolism. They usually occur as a result of a myxoma in the left atrium and most commonly affect the middle cerebral artery.[11]

Miliary aneurysms are extremely small and occur on branches of the cerebral arteries in the basal ganglia, thalamus, pons, cerebellum, and cerebral cortex.[12] They are thought to be associated with hypertension and believed to be the cause of many hypertensive cerebral hemorrhages.

Fusiform aneurysms are a general dilatation of the blood vessel on all sides and usually occur in large, severely atherosclerotic and tortuous vessels. Because of chronic bending of the artery, it is thought that transverse tears occur in the internal elastic lamina, affecting the layers in the vessel and ultimately leading to vessel atrophy and weakness against hemodynamic stress.[13]

There are 4 types of aneurysms that occur in association with AVMs: unassociated, proximal, pedicle, and intranidal. Unassociated aneurysms typically occur on the circle of Willis, in a location not associated hemodynamically with the AVM. Proximal aneurysms occur on the proximal vessel that feeds the AVM. Pedicle aneurysms occur along AVM arterial feeders. Intranidal aneurysms occur within the AVM nidus and are often the source of the AVM hemorrhage. It is believed that hemodynamic stress from turbulent high flow states leads to aneurysm formation.[14,15] All aneurysms are considered giant when they measure more than 2.5 cm in diameter.

DIAGNOSIS

Diagnosis of aneurysm and SAH is often made based on clinical presentation and risk factors. Typical presentation of patients with SAH is often associated with a complaint of having the "worst headache of my life," associated nausea and vomiting, neck pain or stiffness, photophobia, and loss of consciousness.[4] Additional findings on physical examination may include retinal hemorrhages, meningismus, and diminished level of consciousness.[4] Localizing neurologic signs may also exist, such as third or sixth nerve palsies, bilateral lower extremity weakness, abulia, hemiparesis with aphasia, or neglect.[4] SAH may be mistaken for migraine or other benign cephalgias and failure to correctly diagnose SAH is associated with worsened prognosis. Misdiagnosis of SAH is common in up to 50% of patients at initial presentation.[4]

A head computed tomography (CT) scan should be the first study that is performed when there is concern for SAH. If the CT scan is of good quality, SAH will be revealed in 100% of cases that are scanned within 12 hours of symptom onset and in 93% that are scanned within 24 hours.[16] If a head CT scan is negative for SAH, a lumbar puncture may be performed looking for xanthochromia, which is best measured by spectrophotometry. If red blood cells (RBCs) are abundant in all tubes, without significant change in the number of RBCs from tube 1 to tube 4, that may also be an indicator of SAH.

If initial studies are negative and there is a high index of suspicion of aneurysm, additional studies may include CT angiography of the brain and neck, magnetic resonance angiography of the brain, and conventional angiography of the cerebral and cervical vessels.

On diagnosis of a cerebral aneurysm, the SAH is graded in terms of its severity. Three scales are commonly used: The Hunt and Hess scale, the Fisher grade, and the World Federation of Neurosurgical Societies classification. These scoring systems are often used in combination when describing the condition of patients and the severity of their hemorrhage. They are detailed in **Tables 1–3**.

MANAGEMENT: A HISTORICAL PERSPECTIVE

The existence of aneurysms and the fact that they could rupture was not described until the eighteenth century. The first surgical intervention was performed by Norman Dott, a pupil of Dr Harvey Cushing, when he introduced wrapping of aneurysms in the 1930s.[17] Aneurysm clips were introduced by Dr Walter Dandy[18] in 1938. The application of microsurgery to aneurysm clipping started in 1972, with the hope of improving

Table 1		
Hunt and Hess severity scoring		
Grade	**Signs and Symptoms**	**Survival**
1	Asymptomatic or minimal headache and slight neck stiffness	70%
2	Moderate to severe headache; neck stiffness; no neurologic deficit except cranial nerve palsy	60%
3	Drowsy; minimal neurologic deficit	50%
4	Stuporous; moderate to severe hemiparesis; possibly early decerebrate rigidity and vegetative disturbances	20%
5	Deep coma; decerebrate rigidity; moribund	10%

Data from Hunt WE, Hess RM. Surgical risk as related to time of intervention in the repair of intracranial aneurysms. J Neurosurg 1968;28(1):14–20.

Table 2	
Fisher grade	
Grade	**Appearance of Hemorrhage**
1	None evident
2	Less than 1 mm thick
3	More than 1 mm thick
4	Any thickness with intraventricular hemorrhage or parenchymal extension

Data from Fisher CM, Kistler JP, Davis JM. Relation of cerebral vasospasm to subarachnoid hemorrhage visualized by computerized tomographic scanning. Neurosurgery 1980;6(1):1–9.

outcomes.[19] Use of triple H therapy (hypertension, hypervolemia, and hemodilution) and trials of nimodipine as treatment for delayed ischemia from vasospasm began in the 1980s.[20,21] Dr Guido Guglielmi[22,23] introduced endovascular coiling as a treatment for aneurysms in 1991. Despite the advances in aneurysm care, death and disability from SAH remain high.

MANAGEMENT: EVOLVING TRENDS AND METHODS

To prevent permanent neurologic disability and death in patients with SAH, today's standard of care comprises many interventions.

Neurologic Interventions

The 2 treatment options for securing ruptured aneurysms today are microvascular neurosurgical clipping and endovascular coiling.[4,18,22] The decision to clip rather than coil an aneurysm is made based on its location, its size, and on the patient's condition.[24] The International Subarachnoid Aneurysm Trial (ISAT) results, first published in 2002 with additional follow-up in 2005, showed that endovascular coiling was more likely to result in independent survival at 1 year than neurosurgical clipping. Rebleeding risk was low, but it was more common after endovascular coiling.[24] There was much controversy and criticism of data following the release of the ISAT preliminary results. Several comparisons were later made, excluding patients who died of rebleeding before treatment. With this change in data analysis, the mortality rate was 6.1% for neurosurgical patients and 6.3% for endovascular patients.[24] All studies done thus far reflect that there are roles for both treatment modalities and that

Table 3		
World Federation of Neurosurgical Societies classification		
Grade	**GCS**	**Focal Neurologic Deficit**
1	15	Absent
2	13–14	Absent
3	13–14	Present
4	7–12	Present or absent
5	<7	Present or absent

Abbreviation: GCS, Glasgow Coma Scale.
Data from Teasdale GM, Drake CG, Hunt W, et al. A universal subarachnoid hemorrhage scale: report of a committee of the World Federation of Neurosurgical Societies. J Neurol Neurosurg Psychiatry 1988;51(11):1457.

deciding which treatment to use should be done cooperatively between surgeon and interventionalist.

Once the aneurysm is secure, monitoring for delayed ischemic deficit due to common complications, such as increased intracranial pressure (ICP), hydrocephalus, and vasospasm, begins.

ICP is monitored by using a fiberoptic monitor, commonly known as an ICP bolt, or by transducing an external ventricular catheter. Increases in cranial pressure occur because of cerebral edema that is associated with vasospasm-induced cerebral ischemia, or they occur because of emergence of hydrocephalus. Treatments for intracranial hypertension include osmotic diuretics, hypertonic saline, cerebrospinal fluid (CSF) diversion, hyperventilation as a temporizing measure, and as a last resort, decompressive craniectomy. Use of brain tissue oxygenation monitoring remains controversial because little is available in the way of randomized controlled trial data, and interpretation of data remains difficult. Brain oximetry data seem to be of limited use as a screening tool for cerebral vasospasm or cerebral infarction after SAH.[25]

Hydrocephalus is most commonly classified as "communicating," in that CSF circulates through the ventricular system, but it is poorly reabsorbed due to blood-clogged arachnoid villa drainage. Communicating hydrocephalus is addressed through CSF diversion, which is usually accomplished via external ventricular drainage in the acute phase, as opposed to a lumbar drain, which carries a higher risk of herniation in the face of elevated ICP. Once patients are past the more acute phase of their aneurysm rupture, a lumbar drain may be placed in an attempt to wean them off CSF diversion, before making a decision to place a more permanent ventriculoperitoneal shunt. CSF diversion also allows providers the opportunity to impact ICP through increased drainage in the face of an acute ICP elevation.

In situations where there is a large amount of intraparenchymal hemorrhage, surgeons may evacuate the hematoma to minimize mass effect and impact on ICP. Depending on the amount of cerebral edema present at the time of evacuation, a decompressive craniectomy may be performed simultaneously with the evacuation. The cranial flap can either be stored in the bone freezer or may be placed in a fat pouch in the patient's abdomen for future reimplantation.

In the case of large volume intraventricular hemorrhage, CSF diversion is critical to facilitating the evacuation of blood from the ventricular system. Once the aneurysm is secure and no further hemorrhages are seen, intraventricular tissue plasminogen activator may be administered to facilitate evacuation of the intraventricular blood. Although there are no randomized controlled trial data to support this practice, its "off-label" use is emerging at many centers, and it may prevent the need for long-term CSF diversion.

Vasospasm remains the most devastating complication of aneurysmal SAH. Assessment for the presence of vasospasm is done using clinical examination, transcranial Doppler (TCD) studies, CT angiography and perfusion, and conventional cerebral angiogram. There are many treatments that are commonly used in neurocritical care units today, and they include hyperdynamic therapy (commonly known as triple H therapy); intra-arterial treatment with drugs such as verapamil and nicardipine; balloon angioplasty; and more recently, intraventricular use of nicardipine.[4,26,27] Nimodipine, a calcium channel antagonist, has been administered as a prophylactic measure that is capable of raising the threshold to ischemia in brain tissue during vasospasm, although it was originally believed to prevent vasospasm. Once vasospasm begins, it may be necessary to put nimodipine on hold because of its hypotensive effects,[28] particularly if hyperdynamic therapy is in use.

Hyperdynamic therapy was initiated in the 1980s, and has since been the mainstay of vasospasm treatment,[29] although no randomized controlled trials exist to confirm its benefit. Animal studies have demonstrated that elevation of mean arterial pressure causes a significant increase of regional cerebral blood flow and brain tissue oxygenation, but that was offset by a reversal of benefit in brain tissue oxygenation, when volume expansion was added to the treatment regimen.[30]

Use of intraventricular administration of nicardipine is emerging as a potentially significant treatment for vasospasm. Randomized controlled trials are still needed, but preliminary data from small case series suggest potential for the suppression and treatment of vasospasm.[26]

More invasive treatment of vasospasm in the form of intra-arterial verapamil, intra-arterial nicardipine, and angioplasty of cerebral vessels is also being used.[4] Study data show that patients with a high risk of infarction from vasospasm who undergo trans-luminal balloon angioplasty (TBA) have a 7% frequency of infarction, which is significantly lower than patients not undergoing TBA.[31] Although there is an inherent risk in performing TBA, the impact in vasospasm reduction is not insignificant. For smaller community-based hospitals, it is the lack of interventional neuroradiology services that prompts rapid transfer of patients with aneurysms to tertiary care centers.

New treatments for vasospasm are being reported in the literature, but they have yet to achieve widespread use; they include clazosentan (an endothelin receptor antagonist), nitric oxide donors, and eicosapentaenoic acid (EPA), an n-3 polyunsaturated fatty acid.[25,32–34] Statins may have a role in the care of patients with SAH, because patients on a statin before their SAH were found to have an 11-fold decrease in risk of developing symptomatic vasospasm.[35] Because of the devastation caused by vasospasm, much research is ongoing in this area.

The development of seizures is of concern, with the need to evaluate the patient for subclinical seizure activity using continuous electroencephalogram and to initiate seizure prophylaxis as indicated.[4] Duration of seizure prophylaxis is provider-dependent, ranging from weeks to months. Seizures occur in approximately one-third of cases.[4] Some studies have associated the use of seizure medications with worse prognosis, although it is unclear whether this was because of the medications or because they were used in patients with a poorer prognosis.[36,37]

Pulmonary Interventions

Pulmonary edema is a common complication of cardiogenic and neurogenic aneurysmal SAH with acute respiratory distress syndrome, and it occurs in 17% to 23% of these patients.[4,38] Use of pulmonary artery catheters was common until recently, but it has now been largely replaced by transthoracic echocardiography and noninvasive Doppler stroke volume calculation, which carries less risk and provides excellent information about forward flow through the cardiac system and overall tolerance of triple H therapy. Distinguishing between cardiogenic and neurogenic pulmonary edema can assist the provider in management and potentially minimize cardiac complications.

During the period of vasospasm, mechanical ventilation is often necessary, given the need for sedation, the multiple angiographic procedures, and the overall clinical status of the patient. Application of positive end expiratory pressure (PEEP) does not appear to impair ICP or regional cerebral blood flow, but it may indirectly affect cerebral perfusion pressure, because of its effect on macrohemodynamic variables in patients with disturbed cerebrovascular autoregulation. If application of PEEP decreases mean arterial pressure, steps should be taken to maintain cerebral perfusion pressure.[39] These pressure goals are typically 60 to 70 mmHg.

Cardiovascular Interventions

Approximately 10% of patients with SAH will have associated left ventricular systolic dysfunction.[40] Rhythm and conduction disturbances are widespread after SAH and can range from fatal ventricular fibrillation to bradycardia.[41] "Myocardial stunning," a phenomenon described in the literature for many years as global hypokinesis and myocardial injury, is theorized to be the result of an excessive release of catecholamines from sympathetic nerves.[40] With most patients being treated with hyperdynamic therapy, cardiac injury is a valid concern, warranting multi-lead continuous ECG monitoring to detect early changes indicating injury, and as indicated, warranting serial enzyme monitoring. Several case reports describe the use of intra-aortic balloon counterpulsation as a method to improve brain and myocardial perfusion simultaneously in patients with myocardial stunning after SAH, but findings from large trials are lacking.

Gastrointestinal Interventions

In patients with aneurysmal SAH, prophylaxis to prevent gastrointestinal bleeding is important, because there is a high incidence of stress ulcers in patients with central nervous system (CNS) insult. Seventeen percent of patients with CNS injury have clinically significant gastrointestinal hemorrhages.[42] No single medication stands superior, but the use of an H_2 blocker or proton pump inhibitor is recommended.

Ideally patients will have enteral nutrition implemented within 72 hours of admission. These patients have a resting metabolic expenditure that is 140% of their normal expenditure, and it often takes a few days to reach goal feedings in this patient group.[43] In the presence of delayed gastric emptying in patients in barbiturate coma or those on paralytic agents, parenteral nutrition is an alternative if caloric needs cannot be met with enteral feedings.[43]

Genitourinary and Renal Interventions

Patients with aneurysmal SAH undergo a large number of imaging studies with intravenous contrast, particularly during the vasospasm period. It has become common practice to use N-acetylcysteine (NAC) or, in some circumstances, a 5% dextrose in water (D5W) and bicarbonate infusion for the prevention of radiocontrast-induced nephropathy. Studies show mixed results about the effectiveness of these treatments, but NAC remains a commonly administered protocol.[44] Serum creatinine must be monitored closely.

Given the impaired level of consciousness in many of these patients, use of an indwelling urinary catheter is common, particularly in the setting of hypervolemia for vasospasm, when intake and output monitoring is critical. An additional benefit of the catheter is the prevention of skin breakdown secondary to incontinence. However, indwelling urinary catheters present a risk of infection and should be removed as soon as possible.

Endocrine Interventions

Metabolic disturbances are common after aneurysmal SAH and include hyper- and hypoglycemia, hyper- and hyponatremia, and disturbances of potassium and calcium. Twenty-eight percent of patients will experience significant electrolyte disturbances.[4]

In addition to the hyperglycemia associated with parenteral nutrition, significant hyperglycemia may be seen following SAH because of the stress release of catecholamines. Hyperglycemia has been shown to increase cerebral edema[43] and is correlated with worse outcomes. Early implementation of an insulin drip with tight glycemic control can positively affect morbidity and mortality. Hypoglycemia must be avoided.

Alterations in the patients' sodium levels is seen frequently, whether as a result of dilution, osmotic therapies, inappropriate secretion of antidiuretic hormone, or cerebral salt wasting. When patients are hemodiluted as part of hyperdynamic therapies, hyponatremia may be seen. Correction with 3% sodium chloride (NaCl) infusion may become necessary, given the relationship of hyponatremia to cerebral edema; fluid restriction is often not used because hypovolemia is associated with cerebral ischemia and worse outcome.[4] When severe hypernatremia occurs as a result of osmotic therapy, diuretic treatment is no longer possible and gentle correction of the sodium level should be undertaken slowly. Correction of hypernatremia can be done by using water boluses via the gastrointestinal tract or by using intravenous solutions, such as 5% dextrose in water and 0.45% normal saline (D5.45NS) or 5% dextrose in water and 0.25% normal saline (D5.25NS).

Musculoskeletal Interventions

Interventions for prevention of contractures secondary to immobility should be attempted as tolerated by ICP. Deep vein thrombosis should be prevented using sequential compression devices and anticoagulation, once the aneurysm has been treated.[4]

Skin Interventions

Because sedation and, at times, induced paralysis is used in patients with SAH, prevention of foot drop and skin breakdown is paramount. Patient repositioning is often minimized because of issues with intracranial hypertension, necessitating the use of special bed technology to reduce the risk of skin breakdown. Passive range of motion, as tolerated by ICP, and protective measures, such as heel-lift boots, circular gel pillows to prevent scalp breakdown, and pressure relief mattresses, should be used.

Infectious Complications

Infection is always a concern, and in patients who are intubated, pneumonia is an almost expected complication. Given the alteration in consciousness that many of the patients experience at the time of aneurysm rupture, aspiration is not uncommon.

Routine ventricular catheter change is not advocated, but in the presence of a positive CSF culture, a new catheter must be placed. A lumbar drain may be an option if the patient is past the more acute phase of injury and intracranial hypertension is not an issue. Urinary catheters and indwelling vascular catheters should always be removed as soon as feasible. In patients receiving continuous heavy sedation or anesthesia, some advocate daily surveillance cultures of blood, urine, sputum, and CSF, because common infectious indicators, such as fever and elevated white blood cell count, may be suppressed by agents such as barbiturates.

Psychosocial Issues

Patients with aneurysmal SAH have prolonged hospital courses, with high morbidity and mortality. Family members need frequent and repetitive education as to the patient's clinical condition, emerging complications, and prognosis. Setting expectations early, of the need for rehabilitation and the potential for developing serious neurologic deficits, can help families prepare for the many life changes that are expected.

PROGNOSIS AND ETHICAL CONSIDERATIONS

Patients with aneurysmal SAH have highly variable outcomes, and predicting functional outcome remains difficult. Morbidity and mortality are influenced by the extent of hemorrhage, the age of the patient, the presence or absence of comorbid conditions, and the occurrence of medical complications. Unfortunately, mortality remains high, with 50% not surviving at 1 year.

Ogilvy and Carter[45] have developed a classification scheme to predict outcome, which uses a point system based on 5 factors: age greater than 50 years; Hunt and Hess grade 4 or 5; Fisher scale 3 or 4; aneurysm size greater than 10 mm; and posterior circulation aneurysm 25 mm or more. It remains to be validated.

Quality-of-life issues are difficult in patients with SAH because many will not have a complete recovery. Conversations need to be held often and early regarding the likelihood of diminished mental and physical capacity following SAH. A patient's advance directives may provide some assistance to family members struggling with decisions regarding patient care. In patients with concurrent multisystem organ failure, deciding between continuation of treatment and withdrawal of care is important, with clear and consistent messages being provided to family members about prognosis and long-term dependency versus complete recovery.

SUMMARY

Patients with SAH may experience a multitude of complications following their hemorrhage. Although their treatment may parallel that of someone with another type of hemorrhage or intracranial injury, there are issues that are specific to the sequelae of SAH and require specific interventions. Treatment for vasospasm remains one of the greatest challenges in aneurysm care.

Patients with SAH are among the most complex of patients with neurologic injury. Brain injury that occurs secondary to vasospasm, and the limited treatments available for vasospasm, make this a challenging diagnosis to treat. Many hospitals are unable to offer all of the services necessary to support SAH, such as TCDs and interventional neuroradiologists, resulting in the need for referral of these patients directly to tertiary care centers for treatment and management. As greater understanding is gained from studies regarding vasospasm, our ability to successfully treat this complication, while preventing secondary ischemic stroke, will improve survival and outcomes.

REFERENCES

1. Keedy A. An overview of intracranial aneurysms. Mcgill J Med 2006;9(2):141–6.
2. van Gijn J, Kerr RS, Rinkel GJ. Subarachnoid haemorrhage. Lancet 2007; 369(9558):306–18.
3. Wardlaw JM, White PM. The detection and management of unruptured intracranial aneurysms. Brain 2000;123(Pt 2):205–21.
4. Suarez JI, Tarr RW, Selman WR. Aneurysmal subarachnoid hemorrhage. N Engl J Med 2006;354(4):387–96.
5. Mayberg MR, Batjer HH, Dacey R, et al. Guidelines for the management of aneurysmal subarachnoid hemorrhage. A statement for healthcare professionals from a special writing group of the Stroke Council, American Heart Association. Circulation 1994;90(5):2592–605.
6. Rinkel GJ, van Gijn J, Wijdicks EF. Subarachnoid hemorrhage without detectable aneurysm. A review of the causes. Stroke 1993;24(9):1403–9.
7. Armin SS, Colohan AR, Zhang JH. Traumatic subarachnoid hemorrhage: our current understanding and its evolution over the past half century. Neurol Res 2006;28(4):445–52.
8. Tindall GT, Cooper PR, Barrow DL. The practice of neurosurgery. Baltimore (MD): Williams & Wilkins; 1996.

9. Molinari GF, Smith L, Goldstein MN, et al. Pathogenesis of cerebral mycotic aneurysms. Neurology 1973;23(4):325–32.

10. Yamaura A. [Intracranial arterial dissections]. Jpn Circ J 1993;57(Suppl):41317–8 [in Japanese].

11. Burton C, Johnston J. Multiple cerebral aneurysms and cardiac myxoma. N Engl J Med 1970;282(1):35–6.

12. Fisher CM. Cerebral miliary aneurysms in hypertension. Am J Pathol 1972;66(2):313–30.

13. Stehbens WE. Flow in glass models of arterial bifurcations and berry aneurysms at low Reynolds numbers. Q J Exp Physiol Cogn Med Sci 1975;60(3):181–92.

14. Kondziolka D, Nixon BJ, Lasjaunias P, et al. Cerebral arteriovenous malformations with associated arterial aneurysms: hemodynamic and therapeutic considerations. Can J Neurol Sci 1988;15(2):130–4.

15. Miyasaka K, Wolpert SM, Prager RJ. The association of cerebral aneurysms, infundibula, and intracranial arteriovenous malformations. Stroke 1982;13(2):196–203.

16. Sames TA, Storrow AB, Finkelstein JA, et al. Sensitivity of new-generation computed tomography in subarachnoid hemorrhage. Acad Emerg Med 1996;3(1):16–20.

17. Todd NV, Howie JE, Miller JD. Norman Dott's contribution to aneurysm surgery. J Neurol Neurosurg Psychiatr 1990;53(6):455–8.

18. Dandy WE. Intracranial aneurysm of the internal carotid artery: cured by operation. Ann Surg 1938;107(5):654–9.

19. Krayenbuhl HA, Yasargil MG, Flamm ES, et al. Microsurgical treatment of intracranial saccular aneurysms. J Neurosurg 1972;37(6):678–86.

20. Allen GS, Ahn HS, Preziosi TJ, et al. Cerebral arterial spasm–a controlled trial of nimodipine in patients with subarachnoid hemorrhage. N Engl J Med 1983;308(11):619–24.

21. Pickard JD, Murray GD, Illingworth R, et al. Effect of oral nimodipine on cerebral infarction and outcome after subarachnoid haemorrhage: British aneurysm nimodipine trial. BMJ 1989;298(6674):636–42.

22. Guglielmi G, Vinuela F, Dion J, et al. Electrothrombosis of saccular aneurysms via endovascular approach. Part 2: preliminary clinical experience. J Neurosurg 1991;75(1):8–14.

23. Strother CM. Historical perspective. Electrothrombosis of saccular aneurysms via endovascular approach: part 1 and part 2. AJNR Am J Neuroradiol 2001;22(5):1010–2.

24. Molyneux AJ, Kerr RS, Yu LM, et al. International subarachnoid aneurysm trial (ISAT) of neurosurgical clipping versus endovascular coiling in 2143 patients with ruptured intracranial aneurysms: a randomised comparison of effects on survival, dependency, seizures, rebleeding, subgroups, and aneurysm occlusion. Lancet 2005;366(9488):809–17.

25. Naidech AM, Bendok BR, Ault ML, et al. Monitoring with the Somanetics INVOS 5100C after aneurysmal subarachnoid hemorrhage. Neurocrit Care 2008;9(3):326–31.

26. Goodson K, Lapointe M, Monroe T, et al. Intraventricular nicardipine for refractory cerebral vasospasm after subarachnoid hemorrhage. Neurocrit Care 2008;8(2):247–52.

27. Raabe A, Romner B. Hypervolemia in cerebral vasospasm. J Neurosurg 2006;104(6):994–5.

28. Vergouwen MD, Vermeulen M, Roos YB. Effect of nimodipine on outcome in patients with traumatic subarachnoid haemorrhage: a systematic review. Lancet Neurol 2006;5(12):1029–32.

29. Kassell NF, Peerless SJ, Durward QJ, et al. Treatment of ischemic deficits from vasospasm with intravascular volume expansion and induced arterial hypertension. Neurosurgery 1982;11(3):337–43.
30. Muench E, Horn P, Bauhuf C, et al. Effects of hypervolemia and hypertension on regional cerebral blood flow, intracranial pressure, and brain tissue oxygenation after subarachnoid hemorrhage. Crit Care Med 2007;35(8):1844–51.
31. Jestaedt L, Pham M, Bartsch AJ, et al. The impact of balloon angioplasty on the evolution of vasospasm-related infarction after aneurysmal subarachnoid hemorrhage. Neurosurgery 2008;62(3):610–7.
32. Macdonald RL, Kassell NF, Mayer S, et al. Clazosentan to overcome neurological ischemia and infarction occurring after subarachnoid hemorrhage (CONSCIOUS-1): randomized, double-blind, placebo-controlled phase 2 dose-finding trial. Stroke 2008;39(11):3015–21.
33. Sehba FA, Friedrich V Jr, Makonnen G, et al. Acute cerebral vascular injury after subarachnoid hemorrhage and its prevention by administration of a nitric oxide donor. J Neurosurg 2007;106(2):321–9.
34. Yoneda H, Shirao S, Kurokawa T, et al. Does eicosapentaenoic acid (EPA) inhibit cerebral vasospasm in patients after aneurysmal subarachnoid hemorrhage? Acta Neurol Scand 2008;118(1):54–9.
35. McGirt MJ, Blessing R, Alexander MJ, et al. Risk of cerebral vasospasm after subarachnoid hemorrhage reduced by statin therapy: a multivariate analysis of an institutional experience. J Neurosurg 2006;105(5):671–4.
36. Naidech AM, Kreiter KT, Janjua N, et al. Phenytoin exposure is associated with functional and cognitive disability after subarachnoid hemorrhage. Stroke 2005; 36(3):583–7.
37. Rosengart AJ, Schultheiss KE, Tolentino J, et al. Prognostic factors for outcome in patients with aneurysmal subarachnoid hemorrhage. Stroke 2007;38(8):2315–21.
38. Sen J, Belli A, Albon H, et al. Triple-H therapy in the management of aneurysmal subarachnoid haemorrhage. Lancet Neurol 2003;2(10):614–21.
39. Muench E, Bauhuf C, Roth H, et al. Effects of positive end-expiratory pressure on regional cerebral blood flow, intracranial pressure, and brain tissue oxygenation. Crit Care Med 2005;33(10):2367–72.
40. Banki NM, Kopelnik A, Dae MW, et al. Acute neurocardiogenic injury after subarachnoid hemorrhage. Circulation 2005;112(21):3314–9.
41. Macmillan CS, Grant IS, Andrews PJ. Pulmonary and cardiac sequelae of subarachnoid haemorrhage: time for active management? Intensive Care Med 2002;28(8):1012–23.
42. Lu WY, Rhoney DH, Boling WB, et al. A review of stress ulcer prophylaxis in the neurosurgical intensive care unit. Neurosurgery 1997;41(2):416–25.
43. Greenberg MS. Handbook of neurosurgery. Lakeland (FL): Thieme; 2001.
44. Fishbane S, Durham JH, Marzo K, et al. N-acetylcysteine in the prevention of radiocontrast-induced nephropathy. J Am Soc Nephrol 2004;15(2):251–60.
45. Ogilvy CS, Carter BS. A proposed comprehensive grading system to predict outcome for surgical management of intracranial aneurysms. Neurosurgery 1998;42(5):959–68.

Telestroke: State of the Science and Steps for Implementation

Dana A. Stradling, RN, BSN, CNRN

KEYWORDS

- Stroke • Telemedicine • Telestroke • Nurse • Stroke care
- Stroke management

Stroke is a major public health problem worldwide. It is the number three cause of death in the United States, behind diseases of the heart and cancer, and is the number one cause of adult disability.[1] Direct and indirect costs of stroke are estimated to be $62.7 billion annually in the United States, with 15% to 30% of stroke survivors being permanently disabled and 20% requiring institutional care at 3 months after stroke. Direct costs are attributed to the initial hospitalization, skilled nursing care, physician and nursing care, medications and durable medical equipment, home health care, and acute rehabilitation. Indirect costs include loss of productivity due to morbidity and mortality, and loss of esteem due to disability.[2]

In Western societies, about 80% of strokes occur because of a blockage of an artery in the brain by a clot (thrombosis). The part of the brain that is supplied by the clotted blood vessel is then deprived of blood and oxygen. As a result of the deprived blood and oxygen, the cells of that part of the brain die. This type of stroke is called an ischemic stroke. The remaining 20% are caused by hemorrhages. Given the narrow therapeutic windows for treatment of acute ischemic stroke, timely evaluation and diagnosis of ischemic stroke are paramount.[1]

Rapid recognition and accurate diagnosis are critical to optimize outcomes in patients with acute stroke. A variety of conditions can mimic acute stroke, and the ability to rapidly and accurately differentiate among these can be challenging for the Advanced Practice Nurse (APN) and physician without neurologic expertise. The misdiagnosis rate by primary care and emergency physicians is substantial and may be as high as 30%. Delays in diagnosis, misdiagnosis, and complete failure to diagnose acute stroke limit the use of proven therapies such as the clot-buster drug, tissue plasminogen activator (tPA). Current recommendations and drug labeling limit the use of intravenous (IV) tPA in the United States to within 3 to 4.5 hours of the time the patient was last seen healthy (or had witnessed onset of symptoms).

Case Management, UC Irvine Medical Center, 101 The City Drive, Building 53 Room 225C RT 81, Orange, CA 92868, USA
E-mail address: dstradli@uci.edu

Crit Care Nurs Clin N Am 21 (2009) 541–548
doi:10.1016/j.ccell.2009.07.017
0899-5885/09/$ – see front matter © 2009 Elsevier Inc. All rights reserved.

ccnursing.theclinics.com

Emergency nurses understand that time is critical and are trained in rapid assessment and treatment of stroke patients.[3]

The reversal or reduction of stroke disability depends on timely triage, assessment, and treatment beginning in the prehospital care sector, continuing in the emergency department (ED), and throughout the acute care phase of treatment.[1] One way that this goal can be accomplished is through formation of interdisciplinary stroke teams, which includes nurses trained in stroke and operate based on the idea that "time is brain," providing highly specialized expert care to complex, vulnerable patients. Whether functioning as a staff nurse, APN, nurse manager, or nurse researcher, provision of care to acute stroke patients requires a significant commitment on the part of the nursing profession to ensure timely, expert care delivery, and ongoing performance improvement.[3]

One major challenge is to increase access to appropriate interventions for stroke among patients in remote or underserved regions. Organization of stroke care with proper access to vascular neurology expertise is an important component of stroke prevention, because it provides an opportunity for proper identification of stroke subtype followed by individualized, evidence-based secondary stroke prevention. In many areas of the world, including developed and developing regions, access to vascular neurologists, general neurologists, and nurses with special training in acute stroke treatment and prevention is sorely lacking.[4]

REVIEW OF LITERATURE

Telemedicine or telehealth has been broadly defined as the use of telecommunications technologies to provide medical information and services. The use of telemedicine in the treatment of stroke, commonly referred to as telestroke, has shown great promise in improving patient access to recommended stroke treatments in rural and other "neurologically underserved" areas.[4] Use of interactive full-motion audio and video for acute stroke care was first reported in the early 1990s, but Levine and Gorman[5] were the first to coin the term telestroke for the use of high-quality interactive telemedicine in acute stroke intervention. Over the past 2 decades, this model has been adopted and implemented by multiple different types of health care organizations across the United States and abroad.[6]

Fisher[7] proposed a hub-and-spoke model of telemedicine-delivered stroke care designed to enhance the administration of acute stroke therapies. Evidence-based care from the hub, which should ideally be a Joint Commission–certified Primary Stroke Center, is transmitted to the spokes. Hubs are generally located in urban areas, and spokes are usually located in rural regions or in urban hospitals that are not stroke centers. The optimal telestroke spoke hospital has a sufficient volume of patients with acute stroke but does not have available nurses and physicians with stroke expertise on-call for emergencies.[8]

In 2005, the American Stroke Association formed a task force on the development of stroke systems to propose a new framework for stroke-care delivery that would emphasize linkages rather than silos in the chain of stroke survival, and provide a blueprint for large organizations or state and federal agencies on how to implement a more coordinated approach to stroke care. The stroke systems of care model recommends implementation of telemedicine and aeromedical transport to increase access to acute stroke care in neurologically underserved areas, as do the latest American Stroke Association guidelines for the early management of adults with ischemic stroke.[6]

Telenursing is the use of telecommunications and information technology for providing nursing services in health care to enhance care whenever a physical distance exists between patient and nurse or between any number of nurses.[9] Telestroke services that telenurses provide include, but are not limited to, stroke health assessment and triage; provision of health information; and health counseling and teaching. Using telehealth applications, nurses can extend and share their knowledge and skills. Nurses are integral to an effective, coordinated health care delivery model.[10]

The core steps of an acute stroke clinical encounter include rapid neurologic assessment, review of brain imaging, and clinical formulation. For example, exclusion of stroke mimics and assessment of patient eligibility for thrombolytic therapy (IV tPA), investigational stroke clinical trials, or more advanced stroke services.[11] Telemedicine-enabled acute stroke consultation supports the remote review of transmitted medical images at appropriate resolution with the industry standard DICOM (digital imaging and communications in medicine) digital format, established in 1982 by the American College of Radiology and the National Electric Manufacturers Association.[6]

A clinical evaluation is performed over interactive full-motion integrated video and audio (videoconferencing) with common industry standards for far-end camera control, video transmission, and compression such as MPEG (Motion Picture Experts Group) and CIF (common intermediate format) to define resolution and frame rates of projection. Audio transmission incorporates algorithms to reduce the echo and distortion that are common to medical environments.[6]

The ED nurse plays a vital role in facilitating these steps and providing specialists with the data necessary to assist clinicians at the bedside in stroke-related decision-making for patients presenting at distant or underequipped facilities. Nurses assist the physicians in the implementation of acute stroke treatment protocols and coordinating connections between remote sites. Telestroke nurses are critical in first point of contact for patients presenting to the ED. When a patient presents with signs and symptoms of stroke, the ED nurses activate the stroke code protocol, which includes the activating the telestroke hotline at the hub site.[6]

The nurse must first determine when stroke symptoms began; this information is key in determining the course of care. The ED nurse and physician work as a team to quickly complete a history physical assessment, electrocardiogram, IV access, and blood collection in preparation for timely transport to the CT scan. Nurses also determine the severity of stroke symptoms using the National Institutes of Health Stroke Scale (NIHSS). Based on this information, the hub physician can offer a definitive expert opinion on the correct diagnosis and most advisable treatment plan. Management recommendations may include supportive care, additional diagnostic tests, and thrombolytic therapy.[3]

Telestroke allows a nurse and physician consultation with remote cerebrovascular specialists from virtually any location within minutes of attempted contact, enhancing the care of any individual patient.[12] It also facilitates the stroke research nurse to enhance patient entry into stroke clinical trials. Nursing research coordinators responsible for the screening, enrollment of patients into medical trials, and ongoing patient management and evaluation are common to comprehensive stroke centers, fostering conduct of exciting experimental studies aimed at reducing stroke disability.[3]

Beginning with a patient's early recognition of stroke symptoms and culminating in a successful telestroke consultation, each step along the way is crucial to the outcome. **Table 1** depicts possible steps and target times for the telestroke chain of survival. The spoke emergency physician performs a quick assessment, recognizes an acute stroke syndrome, and activates the telestroke hotline at the hub site. Developing an algorithm for the step-by-step conduct of a telestroke consultation is important to developing a telestroke standard of care. In ideal practice, the spoke and hub

Table 1
Suggested target intervals (from ED arrival to activity) for a telestroke consultation

Activity	Time (min)
Emergency department arrival	0
Triage nurse assessment	5
Emergency physician assessment	10
Laboratory tests and CT of head ordered	15
Laboratory tests and CT of head conducted	25
Telestroke hotline activated by spoke hospital	30
Preliminary telephone communication between hub and spoke hospitals	35
2-way audiovisual telestroke consultation commences	40
Teleradiology review of head CT	45
Diagnosis of stroke established and eligibility for short-term treatment determined	55
Treatments recommended and administered	60
Admission or transfer arranged, marking end of telestroke consultation	65
Consultation note dictated by hub hospital neurologist	75
Consultation note transcribed and transmitted to spoke hospital	120

centers should use the same stroke alert algorithm to create continuity of care throughout an acute stroke evaluation.[13]

Telestroke is a subcategory of the drip-and-ship design. Drip-and-ship describes the treatment of acute ischemic stroke patients with IV tPA in a community ED followed by transfer to a comprehensive stroke center. Typically, the decision regarding tPA administration is made by a local physician in the referring center in telephone consultation with a stroke specialist. Critical determining factors for treatment, such as time of onset, blood pressure, neurologic examination, and CT findings, are determined by the local physician. Transportation to the tertiary center is by ground or air, often while the tPA is still infusing. Following arrival at the tertiary center, the patient may be reassessed for potential benefit from intra-arterial therapies.

The drip-and-ship method for delivering acute stroke therapy increases the number of patients who may benefit from IV tPA. Patient selection for IV tPA with the drip-and-ship approach involves a discussion between an emergency physician at the local hospital and a stroke physician at the hub.[14] **Box 1** illustrates an example of an emergency medical service (EMS) post-IV tPA transfer protocol from Massachusetts General Hospital.[15]

DISCUSSION ON THE POTENTIAL IMPACT

There are a growing number of telestroke programs established in the United States and Europe. These range from small partnerships between individual campuses of a single hospital system to large multihospital affiliations in which nonprofit, academic medical centers or tertiary hospitals serve as the hubs to a network of spokes. The reported numbers of telestroke consultations overall, and those that lead to thrombolysis, show that the use of telemedicine is feasible and has already affected local stroke care.[7]

The telestroke centers have convincingly demonstrated the feasibility and reliability of performing validated clinical stroke severity scales by nurses and physicians, and supervising the remote administration of IV tPA by use of telestroke, which has

Box 1
EMS post-IV tPA transfer protocol from Massachusetts General Hospital

All post-tPA patients should be sent by critical care transport or by ALS with the following instructions:

Document vital signs before transport and verify that SBP < 180, DBP< 105. If BP above limits, sending hospital should stabilize before transport

Obtain contact method for family or caregiver (preferably cell phone) to allow contact during transport or upon patient arrival

Perform and document initial neurologic examination

   Perform and record the Boston Stroke Scale (BOSS) per EMS guidelines

   Perform and record GCS and pupil examination

Continuous pulse oximetry monitoring, apply oxygen by nasal canula or mask to maintain oxygen saturation > 92%

Continuous cardiac monitoring. Call medical control if hemodynamically unstable or symptoms due to tachycardia or bradycardia

Keep strict NPO including medications

Verify total dose and time of IV tPA bolus (if dose is completed before transfer)

If IV tPA dose administration will continue en route, verify estimated time of completion. Verify with the sending hospital that the excess tPA has been withdrawn from the tPA bottle and wasted, so that the tPA bottle will be empty when the full dose is finished infusing. For example, if the total dose is 70 mg, then there would be an extra 30 cc that has been withdrawn and wasted since a 100 mg bottle of tPA contains 100 cc of fluid when reconstituted. In addition, the sending hospital should apply a label to the bottle with the amount of fluid that should be in the bottle (so, if there is a problem with the pump en route the correct dosage is noted).

When pump alarms "no flow above" to signify that the bottle is empty, there is still some tPA left in the tubing that must be infused. Remove the IV tubing connector from the Activase bottle and attach it to a newly spiked bag of 0.9% NS and restart the infusion. The pump will stop automatically when the preset volume has been infused.

Monitor and document vital signs every 15 minutes

If SBP>180 or DBP>105, and if intravenous antihypertensive medication started at sending facility, then adjust as follows:

   If Labetalol IV drip started at the sending hospital, increase by 2 mg/min every 10 minutes (to a maximum of 8 mg/min) until 33SBP<180 and/or DBP<105. If SBP<140 or DBP<80 or HR<60, turn off drip and call medical control for further instructions.

   If nicardipine IV drip was started at the sending hospital, may increase dose by 2.5 mg/hr every 5 minutes to maximum of 15 mg/hr until WSBP<180 and DBP<105; If SBP<140 or DBP<80 or HR<60, turn off drip and call medical control for further Instructions.

   If no continuous infusion, then give metoprolol - 5 mg IV bolus, repeat q5 min for a maximum of 20mgs. Hold if SBP<140 or DBP<80 HR<60

For any acute worsening of neurologic condition, or if patient develops severe headache, acute hypertension, nausea, or vomiting (suggestive of intracerebral hemorrhage):

   Discontinue tPA infusion (if still being administered)

   Call medical control for further instructions including decision to adjust blood pressure medications or divert to nearest hospital.

   Continue to monitor vital signs and neurologic examination every 15 minutes

   Contact the receiving hospital ED with an update and estimated time of arrival for all stroke patients, call CMED with entry note when 10 min from the receiving hospital

Abbreviations: ALS, advanced life support; BP, blood pressure; CMED, call medical control; DBP, diastolic blood pressure; GCS, glasgow coma scale; HR, heart rate; NPO, nothing by mouth; NS, normal saline; SBP, systolic blood pressure.

resulted in thousands of acute stroke evaluations and significantly increased numbers of tPA administrations. However, its use must be extended substantially to have a meaningful impact on reducing the burden of stroke disability in our society.[7]

Nurses are extremely involved in helping to establish guidelines and policies for telehealth programs such as telestroke. Nurses provide insights for development and improvement of technologies to meet the needs and demands of the health care providers and consumers. They also participate in development and implementation of competencies necessary for safe and effective delivery of telehealth and telestroke nursing.[16]

Collaboration with developers of information technology systems that ensure privacy and security of health information, while ensuring ease of use and proper information sharing capabilities, is a key function of the telehealth nurse. Promoting the active role of nurses in telehealth includes collaboration with the American Telemedicine Association, their Special Interest Groups, and other health care agencies, organizations, and service providers.[6]

Community education is vital to the achievement of improved outcomes for acute stroke patients. Nurses involved with community outreach may be less available or effective in small or remote communities that have fewer resources. Remote clinical assessment has the potential to be of use in primary prevention of stroke.[17] Currently, risk factors for stroke such as obesity, diabetes mellitus, and hypertension are increasing, and fewer patients in rural areas receive preventive services such as cholesterol testing.[4]

Telehealth is affected by certain legal, ethical, and regulatory issues of which nurses should be aware. For example, in the United States interstate practice of telenursing requires attending nurses to be licensed to practice in all of the states in which they provide telehealth services. Legal issues such as accountability for practice and the potential for and definition of malpractice are still largely unresolved concerns that are difficult to address.[9]

RECOMMENDATIONS

Nurses involved with telestroke must have knowledge of the ethical and legal issues; advocate for safe and effective use of telehealth technology; serve as well-informed resources for consumers and technology; develop the safe use of technology to meet health care needs; monitor outcomes of care resulting from telehealth nursing practice; and ensure confidentiality and patient privacy in all telehealth encounters.[16]

APNs, physicians, and nurses are important gatekeepers in telemedicine adoption and diffusion, and local health care–provider endorsement is an important prerequisite for the success of telestroke programs. In the Massachusetts and Georgia programs, physician and nurse champions at the hub hospitals engaged key stakeholders and other nurses and physicians to promote the development and ongoing operations of the programs. Although the subject has not been studied in a systematic way, there are indications that spoke hospital physicians and nurses are more likely to become enthusiastic participants in a telestroke program if they play active roles in the implementation of the program at the hospital and if ongoing professional and educational interactions occur among the hub and spoke health care providers.[18]

Smith and colleagues[18] noted that for telemedicine to transform the world of health care as the Internet has transformed the world of commerce, several barriers must be overcome. These include: defining the types of specialties suited to telemedicine; developing acceptable policies relating to the privacy and confidentiality of information exchanged over telemedicine; simplifying the process of requesting and delivering telemedicine consultations while also improving the training and education of the end users; developing financial models for reimbursement of provider time spent on consultation via telemedicine; and gaining acceptance of the practice by patients, providers, and payers.

Studies are needed to define a set of minimum technical quality standards for telestroke. Wherever possible, randomized and controlled trial designs should be used to test the efficacy of telestroke on clinical outcomes, with the recognition that cluster randomization may be an appropriate alternative to randomization of individuals in studies involving multiple sites. Other end points to consider measuring are user satisfaction; pace and rate of technology adoption; and changes in nurse and physician knowledge and behavior. The role of telestroke in facilitating enrollment into stroke clinical trials should be explored Fisher.[7]

SUMMARY

In all areas of telehealth nursing, including all related roles and functions, telestroke nurses are committed to leveraging technology and nursing expertise to provide quality nursing care, to delivering nursing expertise to those who need care, and to improving health and patients' outcomes.[19] Opportunities exist to advance the understanding and practice of telehealth nursing. These include developing and disseminating accurate information about telehealth nursing to all members of the profession and educating members of the profession about opportunities to implement technology into practice so that nursing care can be delivered to a broader array of clients, removing the barriers of distance and time.[16]

Telemedicine for stroke has the promise to become a key revolutionary component of an integrated health care delivery system. It can link rural hospitals and under-resourced urban hospitals with regional acute stroke centers of excellence, enhancing standardized streamlined care throughout a system's care facilities.[18]

Telestroke would also enhance nurse and physician contact with stroke colleagues from around the country and other countries to undertake collaborative protocols and research projects and to improve clinical trial efficiency. Telestroke is a new application for existing technology. Therefore, rigorously designed studies demonstrating validity, accuracy, and reliability of telemedicine for stroke are urgently needed to decide whether this avenue should become widespread in clinical acute stroke care.[6]

REFERENCES

1. Adams HP, Adams RJ, Brott T, et al. Guidelines for the early management of patients with ischemic stroke: a scientific statement from the stroke council of the American stroke association. Stroke 2003;34:1056–83.
2. Demaerschalk BM, Yip TR. Economic benefit of increasing utilization of intravenous tissue plasminogen activator for acute ischemic stroke in the United States. Stroke 2005;36:2500–3.
3. Summers D, Leonard A, Wentworth D, et al. Comprehensive overview of nursing and interdisciplinary care of the acute ischemic stroke patient. A scientific statement from the American Heart Association. Stroke 2009;40:2911–44.
4. Hess DC, Wang S, Gross H, et al. Telestroke: extending stroke expertise into underserved areas. Lancet Neurol 2006;5:275–8.
5. Levine SR, Gorman M. "Telestroke": the application of telemedicine for stroke. Stroke 1999;30:464–9.

6. Schwamm LS, Audebert HJ, Amarenco P, et al. Systems of care. A policy statement from the American heart association recommendations for the implementation of telemedicine within stroke. Stroke 2009;40(7):2635–60.

7. Fisher M. Developing and implementing future stroke therapies: the potential of telemedicine. Ann Neurol 2005;58:666–71.

8. Joint Commission on the Accreditation of Healthcare Organizations. Elements of performance for MS.4.120. In: Hospital accreditation standards: accreditation policies, standards, elements of performance. Available at: http://www.jointcommission.org/CertificationPrograms/PrimaryStrokeCenters/guide_table_contents.html. Accessed July 20, 2009.

9. McGonigle D, Mastrian K. Nursing informatics and the foundation of knowledge. Salsbury (MA): Jones and Bartlett Publishers; 2009.

10. American Nurses Association. Developing telehealth protocols: a blueprint for success. Washington, DC: American Nurses Association; 2001.

11. Morris DL, Rosamond WD, Hinn AR, et al. Time delays in accessing stroke care in the emergency department. Acad Emerg Med 1999;6:218–23.

12. LaMonte MP, Bahouth MN, Pathan HP, et al. Telemedicine for acute stroke: triumphs and pitfalls. Stroke 2003;34:725–8.

13. Demaerschalk BM, Miley ML, Kiernan TJ, et al. Stroke telemedicine. Mayo Clin Proc 2009;84(1):3–4.

14. Switzer JA, Hess DC. Development of regional programs to speed treatment of stroke. Curr Neurol Neurosci Rep 2008;8(1):35–42.

15. Massachusetts General Hospital. Telestroke services and protocols. Available at: http://www2.massgeneral.org/stopstroke/telestroke.aspx. Accessed July 21, 2009.

16. Hutcherson CM. Legal considerations for nurses practicing in a telehealth setting. Online J Issues Nurs 2001. Available at: http://www.nursingworld.org/MainMenuCategories/ANAMarketplace/ANAPeriodicals/OJIN/TableofContents/Volume62001/No3Sept01/LegalConsiderations.aspx. Accessed June 15, 2009.

17. Perednia DA, Allen A. Telemedicine technology and clinical applications. JAMA 1995;273:483–8.

18. Smith A, Bensink M, Armfield N, et al. Telemedicine and rural health care applications. J Postgrad Med 2005;51:286–93.

19. Thede LQ. Overview and summary: telehealth: promise or peril? Online J Issues Nurs 2001. Available at: www.nursingworld.org/MainMenuCategories/ANAMarketplace/ANAPeriodicals/OJIN/TableofContents/Volume62001/No3Sept01/TelehealthOverview.aspx. Accessed June 20, 2009.

Current and Evolving Management of Traumatic Brain Injury

Robin L . Saiki, MSN, RN, ACNP

KEYWORDS

- Traumatic brain injury • Intracranial pressure
- Cerebral edema • Barbiturate • Head trauma

Traumatic brain injury (TBI) is a tremendously expensive public health problem in the United States. It taxes the system in terms of health care use as well as income lost because of long-term disability. TBI remains the leading cause of morbidity and mortality among children and adults ranging from 1 to 44 years of age in the United States.[1] Approximately 5.3 million Americans live with disabilities acquired as a result of TBI.[1] Clearly, TBI is a significant health problem among the youngest persons in modern Western society.

Disability and death occur in TBI as a result of both the initial injury and secondary insults to the brain. Mechanisms producing primary injury range from gun shot wounds and motor vehicle crashes to falls while playing on playground climbing structures. Secondary insults occur from such events as hypoxemia, hyperthermia, hypotension, and intracranial hypertension.[2]

Before the advent of intracranial pressure (ICP) monitoring, little could be done to alter the outcome of severely brain-injured patients. Once ICP monitoring and treatment became standard in the management of TBI, clinicians were able to reduce significantly the damage produced by secondary injury.

This article discuss the pathophysiology of TBI and increased ICP, the consequences and treatment of secondary insults, and strategies for the medical and nursing management of the patient who has TBI.

CLASSIFICATION OF TRAUMATIC BRAIN INJURY

TBI can be classified in many different ways. This article focuses on classification based on mechanism of injury and pathophysiology. Classifying TBI based on mechanism requires an understanding of how specific forces at specific velocities produce predictable patterns of injury.[3] The most common causes of TBI in the United States stem from motor vehicle collisions, falls, assaults, and child abuse.

Department of Neurosurgery, University of Colorado Health Sciences Center, 12631 East 17th Avenue, Box C307, Aurora, CO 8, USA
E-mail address: robin.saiki@uchsc.edu

Crit Care Nurs Clin N Am 21 (2009) 549–559
doi:10.1016/j.ccell.2009.07.009
0899-5885/09/$ – see front matter © 2009 Elsevier Inc. All rights reserved.
ccnursing.theclinics.com

Blunt force to the head or trauma caused by direct cranial impact can be produced by the head striking an object (eg, the ground, a dashboard) or an object (eg, a bat) striking the head. This type of injury can cause focal intracranial or extracranial hemorrhage and edema as well as more diffuse injury. Diffuse shearing of axons with resulting cerebral edema and microhemorrhage most frequently occurs as a result of the movement of the brain within the fixed cranial vault. This movement can result from acceleration-deceleration in which the brain, moving in one direction in a straight line, suddenly comes to an abrupt stop (eg, in a motor vehicle collision). Blunt trauma also can be a consequence of rotational injury to the brain. This type of injury occurs as a result of events that produce rotational movement of the brain about its center of gravity and is seen most commonly in child abuse involving shaking of the victim.

Penetrating injury to the brain is caused most frequently by gun shot wounds or stab wounds, either self inflicted or resulting from assault. The extent of brain injury caused by a gun shot wound depends, in large part, on the type of firearm and ammunition used. The location of the injury also comes into play: the more eloquent the territory affected, the more devastating are the clinical effects. Pathophysiologic effects of penetrating injury to the brain include cerebral contusion or laceration, focal tissue necrosis, hemorrhage from damaged blood vessels, increased ICP from hemorrhage and edema, and herniation caused by a rapidly expanding space-occupying lesion.[4]

TBI can be stratified further into primary or secondary injury. The primary injury occurs at the time of trauma and results from focal brain damage and accompanying edema. The blunt and penetrating injuries described in the previous paragraphs are examples of primary injuries. Secondary injuries to the brain occur in the aftermath of trauma. They are caused by a blood flow–metabolism mismatch and result in ischemia that can lead to infarction. They influence the extent of brain damage and patient outcome significantly by compromising the oxygen and nutrient supply to the brain.[4] Secondary injury to the brain following TBI can be caused by a multitude of problems affecting different organ systems. Examples include hypotension, hyponatremia, increased ICP, seizures, and infection.

PATHOPHYSIOLOGY OF TRAUMATIC BRAIN INJURY AND INCREASED INTRACRANIAL PRESSURE

Successful management of TBI involves prompt and prudent treatment of the initial insult and the prevention of secondary injury. The pathology of the primary injury depends on the mechanism of injury and can be classified further based on the diffuseness of the injury.

Focal injuries include contusion, epidural or subdural hematoma, and intracerebral hematoma. Cerebral contusions are the most commonly seen form of TBI. They often occur in association with other injuries to the brain. Contusions are a bruising on the surface of the brain and can be a consequence of blunt or penetrating trauma. The most common sites at which contusions occur are the frontal and temporal lobes, because of the anatomy of the skull and the direction taken by the body on impact (eg, acceleration-deceleration injuries commonly involve a direct impact in the region of the forehead).[5]

Epidural hematomas occur most often in association with a fracture to the temporal bone which causes damage to the middle meningeal artery and subsequent arterial bleeding between the dura and the skull. Such injuries often cause a rapid accumulation of blood in the extradural space, producing mass effect on the brain that, if left untreated, leads to herniation and death. Subdural hematomas are defined as a venous clot underneath the dura. They can be acute, subacute, or chronic depending on the appearance of blood on the CT and the presentation of symptoms. Subdural hematomas are associated most often with blunt trauma but can be spontaneous. Intracerebral hematoma is defined as blood within the brain parenchyma. It often is surrounded by edema and an ischemic penumbra. In TBI, intracerebral hematoma is seen most commonly with acceleration-deceleration injury resulting in hemorrhage into the frontal and temporal lobes.

More diffuse injury involving the brain following trauma usually is a consequence of diffuse axonal injury. Diffuse axonal injury commonly occurs as a result of rotational acceleration-deceleration injury. In diffuse axonal injury, axons and small vessels become torn as a result of shearing force. This tearing results in widespread damage to neurons and often in small contusions throughout the parenchyma within the deep white matter and brain stem. Clinically, patients who have moderate to severe diffuse axonal injury exhibit coma lasting longer than 6 hours.[5]

INTRACRANIAL PRESSURE

It is impossible to discuss the treatment of TBI without an understanding of the concept of ICP. The cranial vault, comprised of the skull and dura, forms a rigid container for three enclosed components, namely brain, cerebrospinal fluid (CSF), and blood. The maintenance of normal ICP depends on the ability of the contents of the cranial vault to remain completely static or to accommodate to any fluctuations. ICP can accommodate small changes within the cranial vault through the displacement of CSF and dural stretch. Increased ICP occurs when the volume of any of the three components in the cranial vault exceeds the brain's ability to accommodate.[4]

Many different mechanisms can lead to increased ICP. An increased intracranial volume caused by an intracerebral or extracerebral mass such as a tumor, massive trauma with edema, or spontaneous hemorrhage causes increased ICP. Diffuse edema can occur as a result of anoxic states or trauma leading to generalized increased ICP. Elevated venous pressure caused by sinus thrombosis results in increased blood volume in the brain, leading to increased ICP. An increase in the amount of CSF present within the cranial vault as the result of obstruction of flow or absorption also causes increased ICP.[4]

MONITORING INCREASED INTRACRANIAL PRESSURE

According to the Brain Trauma Guidelines, ICP monitoring is indicated in patients who have a Glasgow Coma Scale (GCS) score of less than 9 (after resuscitation) and an abnormal CT scan. It also is suggested in patients who have a normal CT and a GCS score of less than 9 if two of the following criteria are met: (1) age greater than 40 years; (2) abnormal unilateral or bilateral posturing; or (3) systolic blood pressure less than 90 mm Hg.

The main benefit of ICP monitoring is the ability to measure the pressure within the brain directly. This information is especially helpful when the examination is poor or obscured by sedation. ICP monitoring allows the clinician to tailor treatment to maximize cerebral perfusion and to determine whether the therapies being used are effective.

When discussing the management of patients who have TBI and ICP, one must consider the accuracy and utility of ICP monitoring devices. Which type is most accurate? Which is most cost effective? Which is most reliable? Historically, the ventricular catheter has been widely accepted as the most reliable and accurate method for monitoring ICP. This opinion continues to be corroborated by the literature despite advances in technology. Many of the other methods for ICP monitoring (parenchymal, subdural) lack accuracy or the ability to recalibrate or are exorbitantly expensive.[6,7]

Although some practitioners advocate brain tissue oxygen monitoring as helpful in the management of patients who have TBI, there are no data from randomized, controlled trials demonstrating that management using this monitoring modality results in better TBI outcomes.

DIAGNOSIS OF TRAUMATIC BRAIN INJURY

The initial diagnosis of TBI is based on history, with special attention to mechanism of injury, neurologic examination, and GCS score, as well as neuroimaging (most often CT) findings. Obviously, history is a key piece of information used in the diagnosis of TBI. Often, however, especially in cases of abuse, the person giving the history is less than clear or honest about the mechanism of injury. Much can be deduced about the mechanism of injury based purely on imaging and clinical examination findings. In fact, some findings are essentially pathognomonic for certain mechanisms. For instance, the finding of subdural hematomas on imaging coupled with retinal hemorrhages in a child is an indication of child abuse until proven otherwise.[4] The important data to glean from the history include the mechanism (blunt versus penetrating), velocity at impact, and point of impact.[3] If none of this information is available at the time of evaluation, then examination with GCS scale and imaging become paramount.

MANAGEMENT OF TRAUMATIC BRAIN INJURY

The initial and subsequent management of the patient who has TBI depends in large part on the pathology of the injury and the brain's reaction to it. Surgical evacuation of intracranial or extracranial clot almost always is possible but is not always clinically indicated and may not influence outcome favorably.[4] There are multiple different ways in which to manage a patient who has TBI, some of which focus on the primary injury and many of which focus on prevention of secondary injury. Prevention of secondary injury after TBI has been correlated with better outcomes and salvage of viable tissue.[6]

SURGICAL DECISION MAKING IN THE ACUTE TREATMENT OF TRAUMATIC BRAIN INJURY

One of the most pressing decisions to make in the case of an acutely injured patient who has TBI is whether the patient requires urgent surgery. Urgent surgery may be indicated if the patient has a poor examination that correlates with a mass lesion on CT (ie, epidural hematoma). The goal of surgical intervention in the acute phase is to decompress the brain by removing the offending agent (most often blood) and to reduce the risk of secondary injury caused by increased ICP.[8,9] In many cases of TBI, urgent surgery is not indicated. In these cases, depending on the clinical picture, placement of an ICP monitor may be helpful in tailoring treatment strategies.

PREVENTION AND TREATMENT OF SECONDARY INJURY IN TRAUMATIC BRAIN INJURY

As previously stated, the prevention and prompt treatment of secondary injury to the brain following TBI is paramount for long-term outcome.[6] This treatment reduces the likelihood that the patient will have secondary ischemia with resulting worsening morbidity and mortality.

Before any targeted treatment strategies for head trauma are undertaken, it is important for the clinician to start with the basics. It is essential to achieve an adequate airway, ventilation, and circulation before initiating treatment. Without these elements, little else matters. When an adequate airway, ventilation, and circulation are achieved, the focus can shift to assessment and treatment as long as no other life- or limb-threatening injuries are present.

Blood Pressure Management

Adequate blood pressure and oxygenation are obviously important to everyone. In patients who have experienced TBI, they have been shown to be crucial. Hypotension and hypoxia strongly affect outcome following TBI. Episodes of decreased blood pressure and hypoxia correlate strongly with secondary injury to the brain.

An analysis of patients who suffered severe TBI with hypoxia showed that diminished oxygenation strongly was associated with increased morbidity and mortality.[10] In a pre-hospital study of trauma patients, patients who were hypoxemic (defined as arterial oxygen saturation [SaO_2] < 60%) had a 50% mortality rate compared with a 14% mortality rate for patients with adequate oxygenation. All of the survivors in the hypoxemic group were severely disabled.[10]

Hypotension also strongly influences outcome following TBI. A single episode of pre-hospital hypotension (systolic blood pressure < 90 mm Hg) was noted as one of the five most important predictors of outcome, even after adjusting for age, admission GCS score, diagnosis, and pupillary status.[10] Hypotension in the patient who has suffered TBI results in a doubling of the mortality rate and significantly increased morbidity when compared with similar patients without hypotension. In-hospital hypotension seems to have similar effects on morbidity and mortality, although these effects did not prove to be statistically significant for patients who experienced only one event.

Of course, subjecting patients who have suffered TBI to experimental hypotension or hypoxia is unethical. For this reason, there is no Class I evidence supporting these recommendations. It is clear, however, based on the available evidence, that hypotension and hypoxia should be avoided or quickly corrected in patients who have TBI to avoid death or secondary injury. Nursing care should focus on the maintenance of normal oxygenation and systolic blood pressure greater than 90 mm Hg. Care should be taken in the administration of medications that may induce hypotension.

One of the most important problems resulting in secondary injury is increased ICP. Sustained high ICP (>40 mm Hg) leads to reduced cerebral perfusion, resulting in ischemia.[6] Indications for monitoring ICP include severe TBI after resuscitation, a GCS score of 3 to 8 in a salvageable patient, and an abnormal CT scan.[11]

Outcome in severe TBI improves when ICP is maintained at or below 15 to 20 mm Hg.[6] One of the keys is determining whether the patient responds to ICP-lowering measures.[12] There are several different ways in which a clinician can attempt to manage elevated ICP.

Hyperventilation

Hyperventilation (to CO_2 pressure [pCO_2] ≤ 25 mm Hg) in a patient who has increased ICP was considered a mainstay of treatment for more than 20 years. Hyperventilation reduces ICP through cerebral vasoconstriction that subsequently leads to diminished cerebral blood flow (CBF) and ischemia. Although this measure is recommended as a means to "buy time" in the setting of increased ICP, it is not recommended for prophylactic use. In a 1992 study, CBF measured within 24 hours after severe TBI demonstrated a significant reduction in CBF in more than 30% of the patients. If these findings can be generalized to most TBI patients, the widespread use of prolonged hyperventilation could reduce brain tissue perfusion significantly.

In a small group of patients who had severe TBI, outcomes at 6 months were worse in the patients who experienced prolonged (5 days) hyperventilation (to pCO_2 of 25 mm Hg) than in a similar group of patients maintained at a pCO_2 of 35 mm Hg.[13,14]

It is clear that prolonged ischemia-inducing hyperventilation in a brain at risk is detrimental. Little is known, however, regarding the effects on outcome of only short-term hyperventilation. More study is needed on this often-used maneuver. For this reason, the Brain Trauma Guidelines recommend that hyperventilation not be used at all in the first 24 hours after severe TBI, because during this time frame most patients already have a significant decline in CBF.[11]

Steroids

Use of steroids is contraindicated as a means of treating TBI.[15] The scientific basis originally supporting the use of steroids in neurosurgery began with the treatment of cerebral edema, most often in patients who had a brain tumor. Steroids have a variety of effects on injured brain. Most notably, they can restore vascular permeability in patients who have cerebral edema, leading to reduction in cerebral water. Steroids also positively influence the clinical picture in patients who have cerebral edema caused by brain tumors. For these reasons, it became commonplace to administer steroids to patients undergoing neurosurgical procedures, including patients who had TBI.

Early studies testing use of steroids in TBI seemed to support their use.[16] Subsequent trials studying steroids in the treatment of TBI actually demonstrated harmful effects, most notably increased mortality. For instance, one of the most recent and largest studies, the Corticosteroid Randomization After Significant Head Injury (CRASH) trial, demonstrated an increased risk of mortality at 2 weeks in patients treated with steroids versus placebo. This finding remained true even after adjustments were made for other injuries and was not explained as a result of gastrointestinal bleeding or infection.[15]

Hyperosmolar Therapy

Mannitol and hypertonic saline are hyperosmolar therapies often used in the treatment of elevated ICP associated with TBI. Mannitol often is used as a "Band-aid" in brain trauma. In other words, the administration of mannitol buys the clinician precious time in which to perform other diagnostic or therapeutic maneuvers in an effort determine the cause of the problem more definitively.

The mechanism of action of mannitol is not entirely understood. It does exert rheological effects that lead to expansion of plasma with resulting reduction in hematocrit and blood viscosity, and this reduction in turn increases CBF. This mechanism often is cited as the explanation for this drug's ability to lower ICP quickly. Mannitol also produces an osmotic diuresis that persists for several hours after dosing.[17,18] It seems to be most effective when used in single doses as needed rather than as a continuous drip. Past studies have demonstrated mannitol's consistent effectiveness lowering increased ICP in patients who have suffered TBI.

Nursing concerns related to the administration of mannitol should focus on monitoring for complications related to therapy, most notably hypotension and renal failure. Strict input/output records should be maintained, and electrolytes and serum osmolarity should be monitored frequently. Avoiding significant dehydration, especially in patients who have underlying risk factors for renal failure (eg, hypertension, diabetes), is paramount.

Hypertonic saline is becoming more commonplace in the treatment of elevated ICP. Its mechanism of action depends on osmosis of water across the blood–brain barrier, which leads to decreased water in brain tissues. It also seems to improve or at least to maintain hemodynamic parameters such as blood pressure and cerebral perfusion pressure. It is unclear, based on current literature, if hypertonic saline is most effective when administered as a continuous infusion or as single doses. At this time, there is not enough evidence to support the routine use of hypertonic saline as the sole means of controlling ICP in TBI.[19] Furthermore, more studies are needed to determine the relative efficacy of mannitol versus hypertonic saline in the treatment of increased ICP. As with mannitol, nurses should monitor closely the patient's response to treatment, including ICP and electrolytes, and should intervene promptly when necessary.

Sedation/Analgesia

Another option to consider for the treatment of elevated ICP in TBI is sedation and analgesia. The theoretical basis for the use of sedatives and analgesics lies in the thought that reducing pain and agitation is beneficial in the patient who has suffered TBI. The reduction of pain and agitation, in turn, should minimize harmful spikes in ICP resulting from pain and discomfort (eg, as occur with mechanical ventilation).[20] Sedation and analgesia sometimes are used in concert with paralytic agents to help control refractory elevated ICP.

The medications most commonly used for this purpose are morphine sulfate, usually coupled with a benzodiazepine, and propofol. Propofol has recently come into favor in neurosurgery because of its rapid onset and short duration of action. These features are useful in the neurosurgical setting because the drug does not obscure the examination of the patient very long after it has been stopped. It has the added benefit of reducing cerebral metabolism and oxygen consumption. A 1999 study, in which patientes who had suffered TBI were assigned randomly to receive either morphine sulfate or propofol for sedation demonstrated a statistically significant improvement in ICP control after 3 days on a propofol drip.[21] No definitive conclusions were drawn regarding morbidity and mortality, however. Favorable trends were observed in neurologic outcome and mortality in the patients treated with propofol. Unfortunately, it is difficult to draw conclusions from this study because of the small sample size used. The main drawback to propofol is the condition known as the "propofol infusion syndrome," in which patients can develop multisystem organ failure leading to death. This syndrome seems to occur more frequently in patients receiving high-dose infusions or receiving propofol at any infusion dose for longer than 48 hours.[21]

Barbiturates sometimes are used in the treatment of refractory increased ICP in severe TBI. Benefits of barbiturates include a significant and prolonged reduction in ICP. They also have neuroprotective effects stemming from their ability to reduce cerebral metabolism and inhibit neuron excitotoxicity.[22–24] On the other hand, there are definite drawbacks to using barbiturates for ICP control. For one, they completely obliterate the neurologic examination except for the pupil examination, so the clinician must rely on ICP monitoring as the means for evaluating the patient. Another pitfall of barbiturate therapy is the potential for myocardial depression leading to hypotension. This hypotension can result in a precipitous decline in CBF and exacerbate cerebral ischemia. Diligent nursing care and assessment are mandatory for patients receiving barbiturate therapy for increased ICP. The responsibility for continuous monitoring of hemodynamic parameters and making necessary adjustments to vasoactive drips falls entirely on the nurse.

In the late 1980s the use of barbiturates for the treatment of refractory increased ICP in severe TBI was studied. The likelihood of ICP control was greater in patients treated with barbiturates than in those who were not. (s 73,7) In 2004, the Cochrane group reviewed the three known randomized, clinical trials relating to barbiturates. They concluded that there is no available evidence that barbiturates improve outcome in patients who have severe TBI. (s 73, 19) They also believed that barbiturates' propensity to yield hypotension essentially cancelled out any benefits obtained by lowering ICP.

Although sedatives and analgesics are used widely to control increased ICP, there is no definitive randomized, controlled trial evidence to support their usefulness in this regard or to indicate that they positively influence outcome in the patient who has TBI.[25] Furthermore, more research is needed on the effect of newer sedatives (eg, Precedex) on ICP control and outcome in TBI.

Hypothermia

There is no evidence from a randomized, controlled trial supporting the use of hypothermia to improve morbidity or mortality in patients who have TBI. In most studies of prophylactic hypothermia, all-cause mortality was the primary outcome measured. Overall, when reviewing hypothermia studies in TBI, mortality was not significantly different between treatment and control groups, although trends demonstrating more favorable neurologic outcome were noted in treatment-group subjects.[26,27] There also seemed to be a correlation between duration of hypothermia and mortality: treatment with hypothermia for more than 48 hours seemed to be correlated significantly with decreased mortality. Interestingly, the target temperature chosen or rate of rewarming following hypothermia did not seem to have an effect on mortality.

Although ICP management is crucial for a positive outcome in the patient who has TBI, the care of this population is multifaceted. Adequate nutrition, seizure prophylaxis, and deep vein thrombosis (DVT) prophylaxis also are paramount issues that must be addressed when caring for these patients.

Nutrition

It is well documented that, despite their often comatose state, patients who have suffered TBI are hypermetabolic. Data suggest that in this population the expected metabolic expenditure is increased by about 140%.[28,29] There is some evidence demonstrating catastrophic results associated with undernutrition in this population. In one study, a significantly higher mortality rate was noted in patients who were not fed adequately for a 2-week period than in patients who had full caloric replacement by 7 days after injury.[27] Another study suggested the importance of early nutritional replacement by demonstrating fewer infections and complications when patients who had suffered TBI were fed within 1 day after trauma.[28] It seems clear that early and aggressive replacement of calories is imperative in the patient who has sustained a TBI.

When discussing nutrition in the patient who has suffered TBI, it also is important to consider the effects of glycemic control on outcome. In animal models, periods of hyperglycemia have been shown to be detrimental to the injured brain and to aggravate hypoxia. Two studies involving patients who have suffered TBI have shown that there is a correlation between poor glycemic control and adverse outcomes. One of these studies looked at the effects of glucose as related to the clinical course of patients who had moderate to severe TBI. The investigators concluded a serum glucose level greater than 200 mg/dL was associated with a worse neurologic outcome in patients who had severe TBI.[30] The bottom line is that euglycemia should be maintained to prevent worsening of hypoxic injury in patients who have TBI.

Nurses have a pivotal role in ensuring that patients who have TBI achieve and maintain adequate nutrition during their hospitalization. They should advocate for early placement of feeding tubes and initiation of nutrition and should attempt to minimize disruptions in the delivery of nutrition to these patients.

PROPHYLAXIS FOR DEEP VEIN THROMBOSIS

The incidence of venous thromboembolic events in patients who have suffered TBI is relatively high. DVT can lead to pulmonary embolism, which entails a high rate of morbidity and mortality. For this reason, attention has been paid to the prevention of DVT. Of course, the treatment of DVT/pulmonary embolism with anticoagulation can be risky in the neurosurgical population because of recent craniotomy or intracerebral hematoma. It is unclear, based on the current evidence, if there is a significant difference in the ability of mechanical compression (sequential compression devices) and low molecular weight heparin (LMWH) to prevent DVT/pulmonary embolism. Both modes seem to be effective in reducing rates of thromboembolic events, and unfortunately at present there are no firm recommendations regarding when it is safe to commence pharmacologic prophylaxis of DVT following TBI.[11] A 2002 study looking at 150 patients who had TBI showed that DVT prophylaxis with LMWH starting 24 hours after arrival or craniotomy led to reduced rates of DVT in this population.[31] The rate of hematoma progression was 4%, however. This study demonstrated that early prophylaxis does decrease the risk of DVT but may carry the risk of increased intracerebral hematoma.

PREVENTION OF SEIZURE

Prevention of seizures in the patient who has TBI is beneficial. Seizures in the acute phase following TBI can damage already injured brain by leading to increased ICP and decreased oxygen delivery.[32,33] Several risk factors influence whether a patient who has TBI will develop post-traumatic seizures. These risk factors include a GCS score of less than 10, cortical contusion, subdural hematoma, epidural hematoma, intracerebral hematoma, depressed skull fracture, penetrating injury, and seizure within 24 hours of injury.[32] For this reason, it is important to evaluate the risk–benefit ratio when considering which patients should receive prophylactic seizure medications after TBI.

Most of the available literature demonstrates that prophylactic antiepileptic drugs are effective in thwarting early post-traumatic seizures. For instance, a randomized, double-blind, placebo-controlled trial in 1990 studied the effect of phenytoin on early and late post-traumatic seizures. It found a statistically significant reduction in early post-traumatic seizures in patients treated with phenytoin (14.2% vs 3.6%). It also demonstrated that there was no significant decrease in late post-traumatic seizures in patients treated with phenytoin. Also noteworthy was that prevention of early post-traumatic seizures did not alter mortality curves or effect outcome significantly.[32] For this reason, the Brain Trauma Guidelines recommends the prophylactic use of antiepileptic drugs for 1 week following TBI. Much less evidence exists in favor of prophylactic treatment of patients for more than 1 week after TBI.

It also is important to recognize that most of the literature defines seizures as a clinical event, thus failing to account for the nonconvulsive seizures that many patients experience following TBI. More research is needed with continuous EEG monitoring following TBI to obtain a more complete understanding of the problem and to allow more definitive recommendations regarding prophylaxis for early and late post-traumatic seizures. Further research also is needed to evaluate the utility of new-generation antiepileptic drugs in preventing seizures following TBI and their long-term effects on cognition.

SUMMARY

TBI is a devastating and unexpected illness encountered by many Americans every year. The management of the patient who has TBI is evolving constantly as new scientific findings emerge. Although many traditional therapies remain important in the treatment of TBI, newer research consistently provokes changes in the standard of care. The need for meticulous nursing care that focuses both on the patient's physiologic parameters and on the patient and family unit will remain the mainstay of critical care for TBI.

REFERENCES

1. Available at: braintrauma.org. Accessed December, 2008.
2. Nockels RP, Pitts LH. Diagnosis and treatment of head injury. In: James G, editor. Management of the acutely ill neurological patient. New York: Churchill Livingstone; 1993. p. 39–48.
3. Saatman KE, Duhaine AC, Bullock R, et al. Classifications of TBI for targeted therapies. J Neurotrauma 2008;25:719–38.
4. Jallo JI, Narayan RK. Craniocerebral trauma. In: Bradley WG, editor. Neurology in clinical practice. Woburn (MA): Butterworth-Heinemann; 2000. p. 1055–87.
5. McQuillan KA, Thurman PA. Traumatic brain injuries. In: McQuillan KA, Von Rueden KT, Havstock RL, editors. Trauma nursing from resuscitation to rehabilitation. St. Louis (MO): Saunders Elsevier; 2009. p. 448–518.
6. Adams RD, Victor M, Ropper AH. Craniocerebral trauma. In: Victor M, Ropper AH, editors. Principles of neurology. New York: McGraw-Hill; 1997. p. 874–901.
7. Shickner DJ, Young RF. Intracranial pressure monitoring: fiberoptic monitor compared with the ventricular catheter. Surg Neurol 1992;37:251–4.
8. Morgalla MH, Will BE, Roser F, et al. Do long-term results justify decompressive craniectomy after severe traumatic brain injury? J Neurosurg 2008;109:685–90.
9. Chestnut RM, Marshall LF. The role of secondary brain injury in determining outcome from severe head injury. J Trauma 1993;34:216–22.
10. Manley G, Knudson M. Hypotension, hypoxia, and head injury: frequency, duration, and consequences. Arch Surg 2001;136:1118–23.
11. Brain Trauma Foundation. Guidelines for the management of severe traumatic brain injury. J Neurotrauma 2007;24:1–106.
12. Howells T, Elf K, Jones P, et al. Pressure reactivity as a guide in the treatment of cerebral perfusion pressure in patients with brain trauma. J Neurosurg 2005;102: 311–7.
13. Muizelaar JP, Marmarou A, Ward JD, et al. Adverse effects of prolonged hyperventilation in patients with severe head injury: a randomized clinical trial. J Neurosurg 1991;75:731–9.
14. Faupel G, Reulen HJ, Muller D, et al. Double-blind study on the effects of steroids on severe closed head injury. In: Pappius HM, Feindel W, editors. Dynamics of brain edema. New York: Springer-Verlag; 1976. p. 337–43.
15. Roberts I, Yates D, Sandercock P, et al. Effect of intravenous corticosteroids on death within 14 days in 10,008 adults with clinically significant head injury. Lancet 2004;364:1321–8.
16. Gobiet W, Bock WJ, Liesgang J, et al. Treatment of acute cerebral edema with high dose of dexamethasone. In: Berks JWF, Bosch DA, Brock M, editors. Intracranial pressure III. New York: Springer-Verlag; 1976. p. 231–5.
17. Barry KG, Berman AR. Mannitol infusion. Part III. The acute effect of the intravenous infusion of mannitol on blood and plasma volume. N Engl J Med 1961;264: 1085–8.
18. Brown FD, Johns L, Jafar JJ, et al. Detailed monitoring of the effects on mannitol following experimental head injury. J Neurosurg 1979;50:423–32.

19. Zornow MH. Hypertonic saline as a safe and efficacious treatment of intracranial hypertension. J Neurosurg Anesthesiol 1996;8:175–7.
20. Bullock RM, Chestnut RM, Clifton RL, et al. Management and prognosis of severe traumatic brain injury. J Neurotrauma 2000;17:453–627.
21. Kelly PF, Goodale DB, Williams J, et al. Propofol in the treatment of moderate and severe head injury: a randomized, prospective, double-blinded pilot trial. J Neurosurg 1999;90:1042–57.
22. Goodman JC, Valadka AB, Gopinath SP, et al. Lactate and excitatory amino acids measured by microdialysis are decreased by pentobarbital coma in head injured patients. J Neurotrauma 1996;13:549–56.
23. Lobato RD, Sarabia R, Cordobes C, et al. Posttraumatic cerebral hemispheric swelling. Analysis of 55 case studies by CT. J Neurosurg 1988;68:417–23.
24. Eisenberg HM, Frankowski RF, Contant CF, et al. High dose barbiturate control of elevated intracranial pressure in patients with severe head injury. J Neurosurg 1988;69:15–23.
25. Roberts I. Barbiturates for acute traumatic brain injury. The Cochrane Library 1999;(3):D000033.
26. Jiang J, Yu M, Zhu C. Effect of long-term mild hypothermia therapy in patients with severe traumatic brain injury: 1 year follow-up review of 87 cases. J Neurosurg 2000;93:546–9.
27. Qiu WS, Liu WG, Shen H, et al. Therapeutic effect of mild hypothermia on severe traumatic brain injury. Chin J Traumatol 2005;8:27–32.
28. Deutschman CS, Konstantinides FN, Raup S. Physiological and metabolic response to isolated close head injury. Part I: basal metabolic state: correlation of metabolic and physiological parameters with fasting and stressed controls. J Neurosurg 1986;64:89–98.
29. Rapp RP, Young B, Twyman D, et al. The favorable effect of early parenteral feeding on survival in head injured patients. J Neurosurg 1983;58:906–12.
30. Lam AM, Winn HR, Cullen BF, et al. Hyperglycemia and neurological outcome in patients with head injury. J Neurosurg 1991;75:545–51.
31. Norwood SH, McAuley CE, Berne JD. Prospective evaluation of the safety of enoxaparin prophylaxis for venous thromboembolism in patients with intracranial hemorrhagic injuries. Arch Surg 2002;137:696–701.
32. Temkin NR, Dikmen SS, Wilensky AJ, et al. A randomized, double-blind study of phenytoin for the prevention of post-traumatic seizures. N Engl J Med 1990;323:497–502.
33. Yablon SA. Posttraumatic seizures. Arch Phys Med Rehabil 1993;74:983–1001.

The Neuroscience Acute Care Nurse Practitioner: Role Development, Implementation, and Improvement

Susan Yeager, MS, RN, CCRN, ACNP

KEYWORDS

• Acute care nurse practitioner • Role development
• Role implementation • Role orientation • Neuroscience

Changes in society and decreased access to care have driven the nursing profession to evolve creatively. This evolution resulted in the development of the role of the nurse practitioner (NP), successfully integrated in ambulatory settings since the 1960s.[1] With time, additional factors influenced the scope of NP practice. In the early 1990s, factors such as escalating health care costs and increased consumer demands for accountability led to evaluation of and changes in health care delivery.[2]

Health care reform was another factor that increased the scrutiny of medical school education and resident work hours.[3] As a result, hospitals have witnessed a shift of medical student training from tertiary to primary care sites.[2,4,5] Around this same time, legislation was passed that limited resident work hours to 80 per week.[6] These educational and legislative changes resulted in a void in care delivery in the early 1990s the role of acute care nurse practitioner (ACNP) evolved to fill this void. Since that time, studies have demonstrated the ability of ACNPs to provide high-quality, efficient care to patients in a variety of settings.[5,7–17]

With quality data supporting a positive role impact, opportunities for ACNP practice have expanded. For example, in a baseline study of 125 ACNPs, results indicated that practice occurred in tertiary and secondary health care settings[18] in a follow-up study of 384 ACNPs, the role had expanded to include a variety of specialty practice settings, such as step-down units, units without house staff coverage, oncology, transplant, cardiology, and radiology units.[19] By 2005, more than 3500 ACNPs were

Critical Care Trauma and Burn, The Ohio State University Medical Center, 410 West 10th Avenue, Columbus, OH 43210-1228, USA
E-mail address: susan.yeager@osumc.edu

Crit Care Nurs Clin N Am 21 (2009) 561–593
doi:10.1016/j.ccell.2009.07.008
0899-5885/09/$ – see front matter © 2009 Elsevier Inc. All rights reserved.

ccnursing.theclinics.com

certified. In a 5-year longitudinal study from that time, the role had continued to expand from the traditional acute and critical care setting to outside the hospital setting.[20] Currently, 4500 of the nation's 195,000 advanced practice nurses (APNs) are ACNPs with 62% of their care delivered in the hospital setting.[21]

As the numbers and opportunities for ACNPs have increased, the successful integration of these providers into the health care setting has become a greater challenge. With approximately 4500 total ACNPs, role models to assist with this assimilation are scarce, leaving the responsibility of role integration in the hands of novice NPs, hospital administrators, or physician colleagues. With few role models, entrance into the new role can lead to feelings of isolation,[22] disorganization, uncertainty, and insecurity.[23] This article outlines role development, implementation, and evaluation strategies to optimize the transition of neuroscience NPs into the inpatient setting. Although this article focuses specifically on the neuroscience NP, the strategies presented may be applied to assist ACNPs in all inpatient practice settings assume significant roles that enhance patient and hospital outcomes.

THEORETICAL SUPPORT FOR ACTUALIZATION OF THE ROLE OF THE ACUTE CARE NURSE PRACTITIONER

Actualizing the ACNP role should be considered a journey that transcends a novice-to-expert framework. Along the path to optimal role performance, ACNPs commonly encounter challenges that relate to the imposter syndrome and the need to develop skills in change mastery.

Benner Novice-to-expert Model

Literature reports indicate that the first year as an APN is a year of transition.[24] As the APN assimilates the responsibilities of the new role, maximum potential generally is not reached until approximately 5 or more years of practice.[25] Obtaining maximal potential requires the ACNP to progress through the phases from novice to expert. These skill stages were described first in 1977 by Dreyfus and Dreyfus (Dreyfus HL, Dreyfus SE. Uses and abuses of multi-attribute and multi-aspect model of decision making. Unpublished manuscript, Department of Industrial Engineering and Operations Research, University of California at Berkeley, 1977.) and were validated by Benner[26] in 1985.

In Benner's model, novice nurses are beginners who lack an experiential context in which to apply the rules they have been taught. Novices can be directed but tend to be inflexible in the way they provide care.[26] In contrast, the expert nurse has an enormous experiential base on which to draw; this experience affords a deep understanding of the total situation, enabling fluid, flexible, and highly skilled expert care.[26] The major implication of the novice-to-expert model for advanced practice nursing is the claim that many ACNPs go into their advanced training identified as clinical experts. Although these individuals may be clinically proficient or expert bedside providers, they can be expected to perform at a lower skill level or at a novice level when they enter the new ACNP role.[27] Therefore, new ACNPs who previously were experienced practitioners can expect to go from their former expert level to novice as they begin their new roles.

The new neuroscience ACNP may be surprised to realize the uncertainty regarding decision making that may occur with entry into practice. While working in the role of experienced bedside nurse, the ACNP probably collaborated with prescribers to obtain orders for needed interventions, but when the new ACNP is placed in the role of the prescriber, uncertainty often prevails. In a survey of 135 new ACNPs, anxiety related to the increased accountability for care decisions caused second guessing of correct interventions. Respondents felt they consulted more frequently in the first 6 months of practice because of feelings of inadequacy and uncertainty.[28] Dreyfus also noted that performance level decreased when practitioners were subjected to intense scrutiny, whether their own or by another person.[29]

During transition to their new roles, ACNPs frequently are tested in all aspects of their ability, making intense scrutiny likely. Fortunately for the new ACNP, Hamric and Taylor[27] have found that new APNs who possess expert bedside staff nurse knowledge and skills generally transition from the novice to expert phases over a shorter period of time. Acknowledging the need to experience each phase of the Benner framework is the first step toward patiently transitioning to an expert level of performance in the role of a neuroscience ACNP.

Imposter Syndrome

As previously stated, intense scrutiny, both external and internal, is inherent to assuming a new ACNP position. This scrutiny, coupled with a conscious acknowledgment of APN novice-level performance, increases the likelihood that ACNPs will experience self-doubt and feelings of inadequacy. These feelings can result in a phenomenon described as the "imposter syndrome."

In 1978, Clance and Imes[30] coined the phrase "imposter syndrome," which is described as internal thoughts of self-doubt and feelings of intellectual fraudulence.[31] Symptoms associated with this phenomenon include generalized anxiety, lack of self-confidence, depression, and frustration with the inability to meet self-imposed standards.[30,32] These emotions may be sporadic and transient in association with specific events such as a role change or an interaction with an authority figure. If left unchecked, imposter syndrome may lead the individual to avoid certain situations or even to withdraw from the role entirely.

Neuroscience ACNPs may be at particularly high risk for development of imposter syndrome because of the nature of the practice into which they have entered. The neurosciences are among the most challenging specialties to master because of the complex physiologic underpinnings, the heterogeneous clinical presentations and the highly vulnerable aspects of neuroscience medical and nursing management. These factors may further contribute to role stress.

To combat imposter syndrome, ACNPs need to identify its symptoms early and to reflect on the validity of these feelings.[31] Discussions with mentors and peers may ease feelings of self-doubt and enable movement to a position of comfort from which learning can continue to support optimal role performance.[28] Foundational clinical expertise should be obtained during the educational process, but maintaining or developing specialized clinical competence in weak areas is another method to overcome imposter syndrome.[31] Confidence develops over a period of time, as small successes in role performance occur[32]; therefore, patience with the processes associated with growing into the new ACNP role should be encouraged. Finally, understanding that role implementation is aligned with the stages of change will assist ACNPs in anticipating periods when increased scrutiny may occur. Having this knowledge enables the practitioner to anticipate or identify stressful situations before they are likely to occur so that appropriate coping strategies can be implemented.

Change Agent

Although increasing numbers of institutions are benefiting from ACNPs, many others have yet to experience this new role innovation. An innovation can be defined as an "intentional introduction and application within a role, group, or organization...

designed to significantly benefit the individual, the group, or the wider society."[33] In the health care arena, innovations typically are new services or ways of working. The benefits of health care innovations are well known and include improved health, decreased suffering, and enhanced efficiency.

The introduction of an ACNP into a health care environment should be viewed as yet another example of health care innovation. Most new ideas, however, are met with resistance, so ACNPs need to acquire masterful change agency skills to support role actualization. Unfortunately, not all change processes end with positive results. In a 1999 study Kleinpell and Nowell[34] found that 6% of ACNPs left their positions within the first year, citing dissatisfaction with or underutilization in the role as reasons for the exit. Barriers to the adoption of neuroscience ACNPs may include lack of commitment to role implementation, active or passive resistance to role acceptance, and lack of resources to support optimal role performance.[35]

Change, for most individuals, is a difficult and a painful process.[36] Levin's force field analysis model describes change as a state of equilibrium between driving forces and restraining forces. Driving forces are the positive forces that exist to support conscious change. Restraining forces are those that inhibit or oppose change. Identifying both positive influences (solutions) and negative influences (barriers) and overcoming these barriers requires change mastery skills.

Change agents are individuals who facilitate movement toward and acceptance of a new paradigm. Canterucci wrote that there is no model for an ideal change agent but identified five levels of change leaders (**Box 1**).[35] Summarizing his concepts, change agents must have the ability to engage affected individuals to ensure support and commitment. Therefore change agents must have communication skills that include listening to and integrating the opinions and doubts of others into the proposed change. As a change agent, the new ACNP must take into account the existing state of the organization and the values, beliefs, and routines of all individuals and assimilate these conditions into the evolution of the role. Fifteen factors were identified as necessary in successful change agents.[37] These factors can be divided into five broad categories:

1. Identifying objectives
2. Defining roles
3. Providing effective communication
4. Negotiating skills
5. Exhibiting political awareness to enable managing up

Box 1
Levels of change leadership skills

Level I: Accepts need for change and defends and communicates need for change throughout organization to create an open and receptive environment

Level II: Defines and initiates change by identifying points in processes and work habits to leverage change

Level III: Translates the vision into the specific change initiative with redirection of approach in the face of new opportunities

Level IV: Manages complex change through integration of cultural dynamics through facilitation of practical course by balancing current reality with the need for rapid adoption of desired future reality

Level V: Champions change, challenges the status quo by comparing the ideal against the current reality; causes crisis to support dynamic actions and transformational change

Incorporating all these factors will enable the ACNP change agent to understand that there can be more than one right solution and to build consensus by differentiating fact from opinion. The application of these skills creates support for the development of the ACNP role development.

ROLE DEVELOPMENT
Barriers

Identifying organizational values, beliefs, and routines is important to support change. The first step toward promoting sustained change is to identify typical barriers that the ACNP may encounter. A classic article by Sullivan and colleagues in 1978[38] identified five categories of barriers to NP practice: (1) psychological barriers that make NPs hesitant to seek increased responsibility and physicians reluctant to delegate; (2) attitudes of other providers related to use of APNs in expanded roles; (3) the ambiguous legal status of the NP and how this status relates to other providers (ie, physicians) in the organization; (4) organizational structures that focus on maintaining the traditional medical model; and (5) absence of uniform reimbursement processes for NP services. Many of these barriers remain as strongly in place today as when the study was published in 1978.

In a focus group study in the United Kingdom, general practitioners indicated their concerns related to nurses' capabilities in the NP role. Uncertainty related to NP training and education, scope of responsibility, and existing organizational structures were all thought to impede the use of NPs in practice.[39] Lack of ACNP mentorship, followed by the level of ACNPs' preparation, along with a lack of physician, nursing, and administrative leadership support for the role have been credited with unsuccessful integration of ACNPs into practice.[40,41] Failure to understand ACNPs' roles, responsibilities, and purposes also have been cited in more recent literature as factors that impede integration.[40–47] Combined, these factors translate into a lack of understanding of the role, along with inconsistent expectations for role performance that may result in an unrealistic workload when different foci are identified by physicians, administrators, and bedside staff.[2,40,43,45,48] Credentialing also may become a barrier when there is no precedent within the institution for ACNP scope of practice.[42]

Solutions

Despite barriers to ACNP practice implementation, solutions are possible when change processes are used wisely and are accompanied by an ability for self-reflection. A clear understanding of the factors that contributed to ACNP role implementation is important, because this understanding provides a basis of support for the role and its related responsibilities.[49] In many cases, the role was created or expanded to ensure consistency of evidence-based protocol implementation. This consistency is of great importance in programs that use neuroscience NP support for ongoing patient management during operative or interventional procedures and when the training requirements of resident physicians and fellows render them unavailable for patient management. Coordination of multidisciplinary efforts is another reason that often is cited for neuroscience NP implementation, because APNs may be more familiar with hospital and community resources that could benefit neuroscience patients and families. The ability to charge one or more ACNPs with the responsibility of ensuring continuity in care despite changes in resident physician and fellow assignments is another frequently cited benefit, because ACNPs do not rotate monthly to other services.

Early in the process of role implementation, the ACNP must determine which individuals will champion, support, coordinate, and market the use of this new role at both the unit and the institutional level. Knowledge of who supports role implementation, their rationale for implementation of the ACNP role, and an ability to bring the role to life in a manner that is consistent with the role's defined vision and mission are among the most powerful factors for ensuring success.

Negotiation

The next step in successful role transition is the negotiation of a position that matches the strengths and goals of the individual ACNP. Negotiating a collaborative partnership begins with a thorough assessment of the individual's needs in relation to the defined role responsibilities and culture.[50]

ACNPs should engage continuously in self-reflection about personal and professional strengths and weaknesses. Weaknesses may include a lack of expertise in areas of clinical practice that ACNPs should have identified and worked to resolve during their time as students, although the need for expanded clinical education and training often is identified during assumption of a new role.[50] Listing educational experiences, special training, clinical rotations, and mastered procedures in a portfolio serves to highlight strengths that may be attractive to potential employers.[51] Portfolios can contain a resume, examples of scholarly work, skills check-off lists, job descriptions from previous employment, scope of NP practice/state practice acts, and pertinent information on successful billing processes.[51] With these strengths, coupled with a humble and honest assessment of weaknesses and an attitude that embraces the value of life-long learning, ACNP applicants are well positioned to assume new roles within the acute care setting.

A clear understanding of future professional goals and compensation expectations is essential to find a position that will be both personally and professionally rewarding. Compensation factors to consider include base salary, work hours, on-call salary and expectations, available clerical support for the role, and benefits that include release time that enables participation in continuing education, documentation/billing, participation in research, leadership, and/or other important scholarly endeavors. Whether a few hours, a day, or a week each month, negotiation of release time should be identified in advance, before accepting employment. Ten percent of the total work time generally is considered adequate at first (**Box 2**).

Job Description

Cummings[52–54] identified three main themes as necessary for successful role initiation: role definition, support of key players, and planning for and evaluating change. During the interview process, the ACNP should request a copy of the job description. The position must be supported by a clear job and scope-of-practice description, because problematic role initiation has been associated with both unclear role expectations and uncertain reporting structures.[52]

According to a study conducted in Ontario, health care providers' expectations of ACNPs often vary significantly. Physicians were found to value clinical care and care continuity. Administrators expected nursing leadership, including role modeling and education of staff. Staff nurses saw the ACNP as a role that would improve access to care and improve communication between team members while maintaining a strong nursing focus.[40] Clarification of ACNP role expectations and reporting during the interview process is likely to unearth important factors that will influence success, and it often is helpful to expand the interview to include key team members. The ACNP candidate then may assesses accurately whether the position is well suited to the

Box 2
Items to be negotiated
Schedule: Shifts, total hours, weekends, holidays, call hours
Vacation: Total vacation time
Parking: Hospital garage or emergency department passes; payment of parking fees
Professional fees: Certificate of Authority, Certificate to Prescribe, Drug Enforcement Administration, malpractice
Books and journals: Annual allowance to cover costs
Conferences: Payment of registration and travel costs associated with attendance at professional conferences; paid release time for invited lectures
Administrative support: Secretary, billing support personnel, office space, computer/printer/software, file cabinets
Technology support: Personal digital assistant (PDA) loaded with applicable software applications (ie, Epocrates [Epocrates, Inc, www.epocrates.com], PocketBilling [PocketMed LLC, www.pocketmed.com], and other applications).
Business supplies: Provision of scrubs and laboratory coats with laundry services; business cards
Protected academic/administrative time: Minimum of 10% of total work time

candidate's individual clinical strengths, professional goals, and personal attributes. **Box 3** provides an example of an ACNP job description.

Matching Organizational Expectations

The ACNP also needs to reflect on individual strengths. Would the best place of employment after graduation be in an institution where ACNP practice already exists, or is creating a role in a site that is unfamiliar with the ACNP role an achievable goal? Without mentorship, a longer ACNP adjustment and orientation period should be anticipated.[28] Realistically evaluating personal and professional assertiveness, independence, and decisiveness are essential for successful role initiation.[28]

Orientation to the Role of the Acute Care Nurse Practitioner

Once a new position has been assumed, it should be supported by a thoughtful, well organized orientation plan. Even experienced practitioners will likely need a minimum of 3 months before they can practice independently. The literature lacks detailed information about ACNP orientation methods, probably because many ACNPs are the first to assume their roles and experience an "on the job training" approach to orientation. Appendices 1 and 2 provide examples of the author's orientation tools that have successfully guided new ACNPs through the process of assuming a new advanced practice position in acute neuroscience practice.

Phases of learning for neuroscience ACNPs include system, informatics, clinical observations, and clinical management. Key to the successful completion of each of these phases is the need to build professional relationships among team members that are supported by trust and confidence in the ACNP. Without these relationships, ACNPs will be challenged in their ability to navigate effectively through the health care system.[55,56]

Appendix 1 Identifies components of the orientation process that are common to acute neuroscience practitioners. The ACNP also should use orientation time to complete his/her own assessment of organizational/departmental strengths,

---

Box 3
Key components of the description of the Acute Care Nurse Practitioner position

Scope of position/position summary

The NP is responsible for providing health care services to neuroscience patients with a focus on management of inpatient service and consultations and outpatient clinic. The NP enhances and expands the patient care within the medical practice and collaborates with physicians and other clinicians in providing a full scope of patient care. The NP has a collaborating agreement with a practicing licensed physician and performs medical services that have been specifically authorized and directed by the collaborating physician.

Duties and responsibilities

Clinical/patient care: 80% of time

1. Evaluates new and existing patients and assesses the physical and psychosocial status of patients by means of interview, health history, physical examination, laboratory studies, and diagnostic studies.
2. Works in collaboration with a physician in formulating treatment plans for health problems and follow-up.
3. Performs and/or assists with diagnostic and operative procedures as designated by credentialing/privileging agreement.
4. Administers therapeutic measures/obtains specimens as prescribed.
5. Interprets and evaluates findings of studies/tests and schedules diagnostic and operative procedures.
6. Recognizes deviations from normal in the physical, laboratory, and radiographic assessment of patients.
7. Relays appropriate information regarding patient care to the collaborating physician.
8. Recommends prescriptions for medication and blood products based on laboratory results and initiates orders for routine diagnostic and follow-up studies, therapeutic measures, and postdischarge care in accordance with written practice protocols.
9. Initiates appropriate actions to facilitate the implementation of therapeutic plans consistent with the continuing health care needs of patients.
10. Evaluates the quality of care provided and recommends changes for improvement in the delivery of care.
11. Triages patients and provides emergency treatment when appropriate.
12. Dictates or writes patient history, admissions care plans, progress notes, and discharge notes; evaluates new patients and makes changes to the treatment plan for existing patients.
13. Documents and promotes appropriate documentation by the health care team.
14. Dictates follow-up letters to referring physicians with summaries of treatment, patient response, and plan of care.
15. Requests records and written consultations from physicians and other health care professionals to ensure patient care is appropriate.
16. Provides preventative health services for patients (screening, risk assessments, immunizations, and other measures).
17. Evaluates new inpatient consultations and communicates the treatment plan to the primary service.
18. Assists the service in the coordination of discharge plans of neuroscience patients and arranges for subsequent follow-up in clinic or with other health care providers, home care agencies, pharmacies, or referring physicians.

19. Establishes a network of referral sources to serve as clinical resources for the NP, the collaborating physician, and the patient population.

20. Maintains contact with and serves as a consultant to home care agencies.

21. Assists in the management of family dynamics and coping mechanisms during acute and chronic phases of the patient's care.

22. Considers the physical, emotional, social, and economic status and cultural and environmental backgrounds of individuals, families, and communities when providing health care.

23. Assists patients in completing forms documenting disease processes and treatment plans for the purpose of health care insurance and disability coverage.

Administrative: 10% of time

1. Participates in review and revision of practice guidelines and related documents.

2. Ensures that departmental and intradepartmental policies, procedures, and standards of care are maintained and assists in interpreting these protocols to patients and visitors.

3. Acts as a role model and resource person for administrators, staff, and the community.

4. Informs supervisors and/or nurse executive of actual/potential problems that require resolution at the administrative level.

5. Participates in quality improvement activities on an on-going basis.

6. Bills and logs all revenue-producing encounters as directed.

7. Adheres to credential/privilege process to maintain clinical privileges.

Research: 5% of time

1. Participates in multidisciplinary and nursing research activities.

2. Applies current concepts and findings from research and studies to practice.

Staff development/education: 5% of time

1. Provides formal and informal education to nursing staff.

2. Participates in development of education materials curriculum, presentations for patients and health care providers.

3. Maintains knowledge of current health care techniques and practices by participating in continuing education opportunities and professional organizations.

4. Acts as a role model for nursing staff in appearance, demeanor, and actions.

weaknesses, opportunities, and threats and to develop an understanding of important political dynamics among team members.[52] The experienced ACNP also should use this time to demonstrate his/her expertise in a humble, approachable manner and to educate informally others about the role and how to best use this new position.

The new ACNP's clinical strengths and knowledge base should be weighed against all components of the orientation, so that an individualized approach may be developed with appropriate time allocated to each orientation element. An ACNP self-efficacy questionnaire, such as the one developed by Shah and colleagues,[57] may be useful to determine how orientation time should be divided among competing priorities. ACNP knowledge should be supplemented continuously, regardless of the level of expertise, so the addition of experiences such as operating room observations, simulation laboratory check-offs, assigned reading, or standing lecture forums (resident conferences, neuroimaging rounds, grand rounds, and other forums) can also be considered.

Methods that support standardization of care, such as protocols, care algorithms, electronic order entry slates, or preprinted order sets also facilitate the new ACNP's learning. For an experienced ACNP who is a new hire to the institution, these structured care methods also enable an assessment of the evidence-base supporting the institution's practices.

A significant amount of learning must occur to support a new ACNP role, but this process must be accompanied by the ACNP's commitment to self-reflection and continuous improvement as well as by clear, consistent, and honest feedback about progress made toward achieving critical orientation milestones. An ongoing frank evaluation and discussion of strengths and weaknesses should be maintained, with clear expectations about improvements necessary to fulfill role demands. Because neuroscience ACNPs rank among the scarcest of NP roles, institutions may be forced to hire NPs who lack a neuroscience background, thereby lengthening orientation times. Although progress must be articulated clearly between mentor and mentee, these discussions must be framed by the realization that entry into the specialty practice of neuroscience is no easy endeavor.

A number of orientation resources are available to assist NPs with entry into practice or transition into a new specialty area (**Box 4**). These resources include national/local organizations, Web-based or book learning, and the use of institutional experts. Membership in a local or national group will provide access to practice guidelines, journals, and social networks that will supplement learning continually. Web-based learning, such as the NET SMART – APN postgraduate academic fellowship program, enables practitioners to access neurovascular knowledge at all hours and to complete their education in a self-paced manner. Interdisciplinary colleagues also may be able to point new NPs toward ongoing learning opportunities. Active solicitation of support from other APNs will help establish good communication patterns and a network of support for the role. Participation in the Advanced Nursing Practice in Acute and Critical Care listserv may increase role networking and support identification of solutions to common practice and professional issues that arise. Finally, participation in institutional APN councils provides a mechanism for discussing pertinent issues concerning advanced nursing practice and evidence-based interdisciplinary patient management.

Initiation of the Role

In studies of ACNP barriers, fostering acceptance of the NP role among nurses was identified as a difficult challenge.[41,58] In one study, nursing resentment was noted to be more common than medical resistance, with nursing non-cooperation associated with fear and distrust of NP roles.[45] In teaching facilities, nurses are accustomed to a model in which interns and residents are the first line of communication regarding patient care issues. In this situation, nurses need reassurance that their role in patient care is valued, and this reassurance may necessitate renegotiation of professional relationships. Having discussions that acknowledge the bedside staff's expertise, while highlighting the ACNP's specialized knowledge, may lessen tension between nursing roles.

During orientation, the ACNP should evaluate the institutional and service line needs to determine voids in care. The interdisciplinary practitioners' expectations regarding the ACNP role should be made known so that clarification of responsibilities can be provided early in a variety of forums, such as staff meetings, resident conferences, and medical service line meetings.[56] As clarity about the role improves, bedside staff, interdisciplinary team members, and physicians will be able to convey the role of the

---

Box 4
List of resources for the Neuroscience Advanced Practice Nurse

☐ American Stroke Association guidelines for acute ischemic stroke, spontaneous intracerebral hemorrhage, subarachnoid hemorrhage, and stroke systems of care; available on-line via free download from the *Stroke* journal Web site; available at: http://www. americanheart.org/presenter.jhtml?identifier-3004586.

☐ AccessMedicine: clinical resource with access to more than 40 online books; available at: http://accessmedicine.com

☐ AccessSurgery: clinical resource with access to online surgical textbooks; available at: http://accesssurgery.com

☐ American Association of Critical Care Nurses; available at: http://www.aacn.org

☐ American Association of Neurologic Nurses; available at: http://www.aann.org

☐ American Association of Nurse Practitioners; available at: http://www.aanp.org

☐ Congress of Neurologic Surgeons; available at: http://www.neurosurgeon.org

☐ Drug Enforcement Administration (DEA) Web site; available at: http://www.dea.gov/pubs/csa.html

☐ *Handbook of Neurosurgery*, 6th edition by Mark S. Greenberg (Thieme New York): a succinct review of neurosurgery diagnosis/literature review, and treatment options

☐ Mosby Nursing Skills; available at: http://www.nursingskills.com

☐ NET SMART Post-Graduate Neurovascular Fellowship Program: neurovascular education and training in stroke management and acute reperfusion therapies); available at: www. netsmart-stroke.com

☐ NeuroCritical Care Society; available at: http://www.neurocriticalcare.org

☐ North American Spine Society; available at: http://www.spine.org

☐ Society of Critical Care Medicine; available at: http://www.sccm.org

☐ State Board of Nursing; available at: http://www.nursing.ohio.gov

☐ Up to date: clinical resource; available at: http://www.uptodate.com

☐ The World Federation of Neuroscience Nursing; available at: http://www.wfnn.nu

---

ACNP clearly to patients, families, and consultant staff. Ongoing education of rotating residents, medical students, and interns also should be considered to maintain clarity about the ACNP's role.[59]

Credentialing/Privileging

Each institution's credentialing and privileging process should be assessed in relation to ACNP scope of practice. Although each ACNP's educational preparation and state/national guidelines play a part in determining what ACNPs may be allowed to do in their roles, institutional politics also may be intertwined in the credentialing/privileging process. Some institutions may offer fairly liberal privileges, but others may limit the ACNP's role tightly. Factors contributing to credentialing/privileging policy may include the need to balance ACNP practice with the learning needs of other practitioners (eg, interns and residents), previous negative or positive experiences with NPs or physician assistants, limited physician resources, the needs of the nursing services (ie, Magnet readiness), and even the need to increase physician and hospital profitability by handing off all medical management to ACNPs so that physicians are free to perform a larger number of surgical interventions.[60]

Consistency and control can ensure quality and safety for consumers but also may impede professionals who have the advanced knowledge and skill to meet the evolving needs of society.[61] As they undertake their role, ACNPs must be knowledgeable about regulations for licensure and about national, state, and institution requirements. Certifying organizations and state boards of nursing should be consulted when questions arise regarding ACNP scope of practice.

For all ACNPs, credentialing is necessary for practice within an institutional setting. Hospitals typically delegate credentialing and privileging processes to a group of peers. The rationale being that peers are best suited to assess the education, competency, and experience of an applicant. Credentialing recognizes the professional and technical competence of a licensed provider.[62] The credentialing committee evaluates the required paperwork and recommends that the ACNP be permitted to perform specific patient-care activities. Admission and discharge activities, prescriptive authority, and procedures are among the activities assigned to most ACNPs, but hospitals vary in the specific requirements and exact processes for credentialing.

In a longitudinal study completed by Kleinpell,[20] 69% to 83% of ACNPs received credentialing and privileging from the medical staff office, 8% to 12% through the nursing department, and 2% to 4% through the human resource department. Before (ideally) or shortly after starting at an institution, practitioners should obtain a packet that outlines the requirements for credentialing submission. Generally these requirements include proof of education; requested privileges; proof of state licensure; standard care arrangements (if required by the state); certification (if required by the state); resume or curriculum vitae; professional references; procedure logs; training records for basic life support and advanced cardiac life support (as appropriate); and procedures requested for credentialing with associated quality-monitoring plans.[61] Once approved by the credentialing committee, the practitioner must maintain institution-specific records for quality monitoring. If no guidelines for an ACNP process have been established, the ACNP should begin with the physician credentialing process.

Procedural competence can be difficult for neuroscience NPs to achieve and should be discussed with the sponsoring physician(s) and administrative staff. For NPs working in a neurosurgery role, desired credentialing items may include such skills as fiducial placement, shunt reprogramming, ventriculostomy insertion, and lumbar drain placement. NPs working in a neurovascular position may be expected to classify stroke pathogenic mechanisms, independently interpret neuroimaging, clinically localize stroke symptoms to discreet neurovascular territories, and, ultimately, to make an independent decision regarding tissue plasminogen activator (tPA) treatment. ACNPs should determine with their physician colleagues what procedures are expected in their role; once the list is identified, establishing how the skill will be learned, evaluated, and maintained is important.

ACNPs who are the first to be hired into neuroscience NP positions in an institution will need to research and develop education and clinical skills check-off materials for procedures. Determining if skills check-offs will be completed in simulation or overseen on actual patients is the next step. The NET SMART – APN program (www.netsmart-stroke.com) requires that a specific number of procedures be performed for neurovascular clinical skills check-offs and includes forms to be signed by the supervising physicians. These forms may be submitted in support of credentialing within the local institution. Other than NET SMART – APN, there are no national guidelines that stipulate the number of procedures that must be witnessed to ensure competent performance for specific neurologic skills. Instead these requirements usually are set by local credentialing committees or can be bench marked against resident/physicians standards. ACNPs working in the neurosciences may need to negotiate methods for the evaluation and documentation of successful skill performance baseline and case logs of credentialed skills performed including tracking of, medical record numbers and complications. Once the minimum number of procedures has been achieved, the ACNP should request permission from the credentialing board to perform a given task independently.

Although procedures are an important part of ensuring timely access to interventions, ACNPs should not fret if performing these procedures is not considered a part of their practice. As outlined in Kleinpell's[20] study of practice, educating patients/families and discussing the plan of care, ordering laboratory and radiological tests and interpreting the results, initiating consultations, and initiating discharge planning remain the five most frequently performed ACNP activities, not invasive procedures. Similar findings also were reported by Rosenfeld.[3]

ROLE IMPROVEMENT
Measuring Role Impact: Outcome Analysis

After implementation, continual evaluation of the ACNP role is necessary to assure that the position optimally served the needs of patients, interdisciplinary providers, and the system at large. Evaluation should occur formally and informally, encompassing both process and outcome components. ACNPs should develop relationships with interdisciplinary colleagues that promote regular sharing of constructive performance feedback. Developing methods capable of quantifying the impact of the role on key patient and hospital outcomes enables the contribution of ACNPs to the institution and department to be recognized.[63] Traditional outcome measures may include length of stay, financial indicators, mortality, complication rates, and patient satisfaction. To establish outcomes that may be specific to the ACNP practice, Kleinpell and Gawlinsky[64] outline five steps:

1. Identify outcome variables that APNs can impact.
2. Organize a team and clarify current knowledge about the practice issues to be improved.
3. Understand sources of practice variation.
4. Select practices and strategies for improvement; plan, and implement according to plan.
5. Check/analyze/review data and results/evaluate effectiveness.

Also key to ensuring optimal role performance is the process of receiving and giving feedback. During orientation, specific time intervals (weekly, monthly, or quarterly) should be established for feedback on specific goals. After orientation, performance feedback should continue to be provided both regularly and on an as-needed basis. Devoting time in staff or physician meetings to a discussion of opportunities for ongoing improvement is recommended to assure ongoing evaluation and enable optimal integration of the ACNP into the neuroscience team.

State or institutional regulations may require that ACNPs regularly submit quality performance data. Beyond these reporting requirements, ACNPs should plan on working collaboratively with information specialists to develop an ACNP "report card" that is capable of quantifying the impact of the role on patient and hospital outcomes. Report card indicators should include core measures for diagnoses managed (eg, stroke, ventilator bundles), as well as metrics that enable standardized assessment of other diagnoses or the development of untoward outcomes associated with acute/critical illness (eg, blood stream infection and urinary tract infection rates). Patient and patient family perceptions of the quality of care should be considered if a system capable of tracking data specific to patients within the care of the ACNP can be established; otherwise, data may not have any linear relationship to overall ACNP performance.

Regardless of the ACNP reporting structure, active participation in pursuit or redesignation of Magnet status should be embraced as a method to showcase the contribution of APNs to hospital quality. ACNPs are well positioned to support the Magnet process by relaying data that reflect the impact of APNs on improved quality of care, sharing the results of demonstration projects that include implementation of evidence-based practice changes, and providing examples of how they have contributed to the generation of knowledge through the conduct and dissemination of original research through professional presentations and publications.

The ACNP annual review should encompass methods that reflect a 360° evaluation of role performance, with contributions provided by interdisciplinary team members as appropriate. The hallmark of a well-conducted formal evaluation process is that the content is already well known to the person being evaluated, rather than a surprise. Evaluation periods should be viewed as a time to acknowledge accomplishments over the previous year and establish goals to direct the next year's activities and as a period of reflection that should enable the recognition of resources needed to support both personal and professional improvement.

LESSONS LEARNED

Those assuming positions as an ACNP often must create their roles, especially in underserved specialties such as the neurosciences. Roadblocks should be expected in the process of rolling out a new ACNP position, requiring a flexible and reflective style that is capable of developing and implementing win:win methods that promote appropriate role enactment. The contribution of many different disciplines to the orientation of neuroscience ACNPs is optimal, because it engages others in the process of sculpting the role while orienting them to the position's responsibilities and accountabilities.

Those assuming ACNP roles must reflect continuously on how to improve their professional and personal contributions in the workplace. Key to this journey is an ability to set appropriate limits on role responsibilities that are in concert with personal philosophic beliefs about the role and future goals. Additionally, ACNPs must commit to quantifying the impact of their role, both to ensure that the value of the role is recognized and to prevent the role's being eliminated during times of economic challenge. It also is imperative for ACNPs to maintain accurate process performance records (ie, procedure numbers and other records.) that are tied to the outcomes that are achieved (ie, complication rates and other outcomes), as well as ongoing education and training records to ensure ongoing credentialing/privileging within their institutions.

The challenge of creating the ACNP role and the journey toward achieving success for the role should not be forgotten. ACNPs have a responsibility to support new practitioners who chose a similar pathway and should regard their new colleagues' successes as a reflection of their own excellent leadership. Finally, all APNs must accept the need for continual, honest self-assessment of their limitations in knowledge and performance; humble acknowledgment of limitations ensures safe practice and provides direction for continual learning.

SUMMARY

A thoughtful approach to the implementation of a neuroscience ACNP role positions these important APNs for success within the health care team. Remaining grounded as a nursing professional while straddling medical practice can be challenging,[55] just as working as neither a bedside nurse nor a physician can lead to feelings of isolation.[55] Accepting these differences while realizing the unique contributions of neuroscience ACNPs strengthens professional vision and enables growth of this key role. ACNPs must recognize that role actualization is a journey that must be supported by humble, honest acceptance of role preparedness that continues throughout the trajectory of one's career, enabling both excellence in role performance and role satisfaction.

ACKNOWLEDGMENT

The author gratefully acknowledges the editorial support of Michele Lindner-Nash, CNP, and Rebecca Coffey, CNP, and thanks Karen Jackson, RN, MS, of The Ohio State University Medical Center for providing job descriptions and checklists. Additionally, the author states her appreciation for the contributions of Karin Grant, CNP, from Riverside Methodist Hospitals and Benjamin Laughton, CRNP, from the University of Maryland Medical Center. Thank you for being driving forces in support of Nurse Practitioner practice.

REFERENCES

1. Daly B. Introduction: a vision for the acute care nurse practitioner role. In: Daly B, editor. The acute care nurse practitioner. New York: Springer Publishing Company, Inc; 1997. p. 1–11.
2. Sidani S, Irvine D. A conceptual framework for evaluating the nurse practitioner role in acute care settings. J Adv Nurs 1999;30(1):58–66.
3. Rosenfeld P, McEvoy M, Glassman K. Measuring practice patterns among acute care nurse practitioners. J Nurs Adm 2003;33(3):159–65.
4. Gaedeke MK, Blount K. Advanced practice nursing in pediatric acute care. Crit Care Nurs Clin North Am 1995;7(1):61–70.
5. Buchanan L. The acute care nursing practitioner in collaborative practice. J Am Acad Nurse Pract 1996;8(1):13–20.
6. Gordon CR, Axelrad A, Alexander JB, et al. Care of critically ill surgical patients using the 80 h Accreditation Council of Graduate Medical Education work-week guidelines: a survey of current strategies. Am Surg 2006;72:497–9.
7. Martin B, Coniglio J. The acute care nurse practitioner in collaborative practice. AACN Clin Issues 1996;7(2):309–14.
8. Hoffman L, Happ M, Scharfenberg C, et al. Perceptions of physicians, nurses, and respiratory therapists about the role of acute care nurse practitioners. Am J Crit Care 2004;13(6):480–8.
9. Kleinpell RM, Ely EW, Grabenkort R. Nurse practitioners and physician assistants in the intensive care unit: an evidence-based review. Crit Care Med 2008;36(10): 2888–97.
10. Spisso J, O'Callaghan C, McKennan M, et al. Improved quality of care and reduction of housestaff workload using trauma nurse practitioners. J Trauma 1990; 30(6):660–5.

11. Gawlinski A, McCloy K, Jesurum J. Measuring outcomes in cardiovascular APN practice. In: Kleinpell R, editor. Outcome assessment in advanced practice nursing. New York: Springer; 2001. p. 131–88.

12. Russell D, VorderBruegge M, Burns S. Effect of an outcomes-managed approach to care of neuroscience patients by acute care nurse practitioners. Am J Crit Care 2002;11(4):353–62.

13. Coitopoulos MG, Mikhail MA, Wennberg PW, et al. A new hospital patient care model for the new millennium: preliminary mayo clinic experience. Arch Intern Med 2002;162:716–8.

14. Burns SM, Earven S. Improving outcomes for mechanically ventilated medical intensive care unit patients using advanced practice nurses: a 6-year experience. Crit Care Nurs Clin North Am 2002;14:231–43.

15. Christmas AB, Reynolds J, Hodges S, et al. Physician extenders impact trauma systems. J Trauma 2005;58:917–20.

16. Meyer SC, Miers LJ. Effect of cardiovascular surgeon and acute care nurse practitioner collaboration on postoperative outcomes. AACN Clin Issues 2005;16: 149–58.

17. Cowen MJ, Shapiro M, Hays RD, et al. The effect of a multidisciplinary hospitalist/physician and advanced practice nurse collaboration on hospital costs. J Nurs Adm 2006;36:79–85.

18. Kleinpell RM. Acute care nurse practitioners: roles and practice profiles. AACN Clin Issues 1997;8:156–62.

19. Kleinpell RM. Reports of role descriptions of acute care nurse practitioner. AACN Clin Issues 1998;9:290–5.

20. Kleinpell, R. Acute care nurse practitioner practice: results of a 5-year longitudinal study. Am J Crit Care 2005;14(3): 211–21.

21. Kleinpell RM, Goolsby MJ. American Academy of Nurse Practitioner National Nurse Practitioner Sample Survey: focus on acute care. J Am Acad Nurse Pract 2006;18:393–4.

22. Koelbel P, Fuller S, Misener T. Job satisfaction of nurse practitioners: an analysis using Herzberg's theory. Nurse Pract 1991;16(4):45–56.

23. Hayes E. Helping preceptors mentor the next generation of nurse practitioners. Nurse Pract 1994;19(6):62–6.

24. Brykczynski K. Role development of the advanced practice nurse. In: Hamric AB, Spross JA, Hanson CM, editors. Advanced nursing practice: an integrative approach. Philadelphia: WB Saunders; 1996. p. 79–84.

25. Cooper DM, Sparacino PSA. Acquiring, implementing, and evaluating the clinical nurse specialist role. In: Sparacino PSA, Cooper DM, Minarick PA, editors. The clinical nurse specialist: implementation and impact. Connecticut: Appleton & Lange; 1990. p. 41–75.

26. Benner PE. From novice to expert. Excellence and power in clinical nursing practice. Menlo Park (CA): Addison-Wesley; 1984.

27. Hamric AB, Taylor JW. Role development of the CNS. In: Hamric AB, Spross J, editors. The clinical nurse specialist in theory and practice. 2nd edition. Philadelphia: WB Saunders; 1989. p. 41–82.

28. Lukacs J. Factors in nurse practitioner role adjustment. Nurse Pract 1982;7(3): 21–3, 50.

29. Roberts SJ, Tabloski P, Bova C. Epigenesis of the nurse practitioner role revisited. J Nurs Educ 1997;36(2):67–73.

30. Clance RR, Imes SA. The imposter phenomenon in high achieving women: dynamics and therapeutic intervention. Psychol Psychother Theor Res Pract 1978;15:241–7.

31. Introduction of the imposter syndrome. Available at: http://www.counseling.caltech.edu/articles/The%20Imposter%20Syndrome.htm. Accessed November 18, 2008.
32. Paul S. Implementing an outpatient congestive heart failure clinic: the nurse practitioner role. Heart Lung 1997;26(6):486–91.
33. West JA, Miller NH, Parker KM, et al. A comprehensive management system for heart failure improves clinical outcomes and reduces medical resources. Am J Cardiol 1997;79:58–63.
34. Kleinpell-Nowell R. Longitudinal survey of acute care nurse practitioner practice: year 1. AACN Clin Issues 1999;10:515–20.
35. Recklies D. What makes a good change agent? The manager.org. Available at: http://www.themanager.org/strategy/change_agent.htm. Accessed November 21, 2008.
36. Norton SF, Grady EM. Change agent skills. In: Hamric AB, Spross JA, Hanson CM, editors. Advanced nursing practice: an integrative approach. Philadelphia: WB Saunders; 1996. p. 249–71.
37. Buchanan D, Boddy D. The expertise of the change agent: public performance and backstage activity. New York: Prentice Hall; 1992.
38. Sullivan J, Dachelet C, Sultz H, et al. Overcoming barriers to the employment and utilization of the nurse practitioner. Aust J Polit Hist 1978;68(11):1097–103.
39. Wilson A, Pearson D, Hassey A. Barriers to developing the nurse practitioner role in primary care-the GP perspective. Fam Pract 2002;19(6):641–6.
40. Soeren M, Micevski V. Success indicators and barriers to acute care nurse practitioner role implementation in four Ontario hospitals. AACN Clin Issues 2001; 12(3):424–37.
41. Kelly N, Mathews M. The transition to first position as nurse practitioner. J Nurs Educ 2001;40(4):156–62.
42. Morse C, Brown M. Collaborative practice in the acute care setting. Crit Care Nurs Q 1999;21(4):31–6.
43. Bryant-Lukosius D, DiCenso A, Browne G, et al. Advanced practice nursing roles: development, implementation and evaluation. J Adv Nurs 2004;48(5): 519–29.
44. Dunn K, Nicklin W. The status of advanced nursing roles in Canadian teaching hospitals. Can J Nurs Adm 1995;(Jan-Feb):111–35.
45. Woods L. Implementing advanced practice: identifying the factors that facilitate and inhibit process. J Clin Nurs 1998;7:265–73.
46. Chang KPK, Wong KST. The nurse specialist role in Hong Kong: perceptions of nurse specialists, doctors, and staff nurses. J Adv Nurs 2001;36:36–40.
47. Beal JA, Steven K, Quinn M. Neonatal nurse practitioner role satisfaction. J Perinat Neonatal Nurs 1997;11:65–76.
48. Irvine D, Sidani S, Porter H, et al. Organizational factors influencing nurse practitioners' role implementation in acute care settings. Can J Nurs Leadersh 2000; 13:28–35.
49. Marsden J. Setting up nurse practitioner roles: issues in practice. Br J Nurs 1995; 4(16):948–52.
50. Shapiro D, Rosenberg N. Acute care nurse practitioner collaborative practice negotiation. AACN Clin Issues 2002;13(3):470–8.
51. Herman J, Selph AK, Knox ML, et al. Negotiating skills: empowering the acute care nurse practitioner. In: Kleinpell R, Piano M, editors. Practice issues for the acute care nurse practitioner. New York: Springer Publishing Company; 1998. p. 79–101.

52. Cummings G, Fraser K, Tarlier D. Implementing advanced nurse practitioner roles in acute care: an evaluation of organizational change. J Nurs Adm 2003; 33(3):139–45.
53. King KB, Parrinello KM, Baggs JG. Collaboration and advanced practice nursing. In: Hickey JV, editor. Advanced nursing practice. Philadelphia: Lippincott-Raven; 1996. p. 146–62.
54. Magdic K, Rosenzweig MQ. Advanced practice nursing. Integrating the acute care nurse practitioner into clinical practice: strategies for success. Dimens Crit Care Nurs 1997;16:208–14.
55. Kelso L, Massaro L. Implementation of the acute care nurse practitioner role. AACN Clin Issues 1994;5(3):404–7.
56. Kubala S, Clever L. Acceptance of the nurse practitioner. Am J Nurs 1974;74(3): 451–2.
57. Stupak Shah H, Bruttomesso K, Taylor Sullivan D, et al. An evaluation of the role and practices of the acute-care nurse practitioner. AACN Clin Issues 1997;8(1): 147–55.
58. Genet C, Flatley Brennan P, Ibbotson-Wolff S, et al. Nurse practitioners in teaching hospitals. Nurse Pract 1995;20(9):47–54.
59. Yeager S, Shaw KD, Casavant J, et al. An acute care nurse practitioner model of care for neurosurgical patients. Crit Care Nurse 2006;26(6):57–64.
60. Affara FA. The fundamentals of professional regulation. Int Nurs Rev 1992;39: 113–6.
61. Hravnak M, Baldisseri M. Credentialing and privileging: insights into the process for acute-care nurse practitioners. AACN Clin Issues 1997;8(1):108–15.
62. Kristeller AR. Medical staff: privileging and credentialing. N J Med 1995;92:26–8.
63. Bryers JF, Brunell ML. Demonstrating the value of the advanced practice nurse: an evaluation model. AACN Clin Issues 1998;9:295–305.
64. Kleinpell R, Gawlinski A. Assessing outcomes in advanced practice nursing practice: the use of quality indicators and evidence-based practice. AACN Clin Issues 2005;16(1):43–57.

APPENDIX 1: ORIENTATION CHECKLIST FOR NEUROSCIENCE ACUTE CARE NURSE PRACTITIONERS

Orientation Components	Orientation Content	Date Completed
System		
	Keys	
	Badge	
	Voicemail	
	Safety	
	Skills Day	
	Collaborative agreements	
	DEA/Certificate of Prescribe/Certificate of Authority	
	CPR/ACLS/certifications	
	AACN neurologic card	
	Hospital prescribing packet	
Computer		
	Neuroimaging remote access	
	Billing	
	Medical record documentation:	
	• Nursing records	
	• Physician records	
	• Order entry	
	• Laboratory data	
	• Electronic discharge tutorial	
Observations		
	Staff RN Neurosurgical Floor	
	Staff RN Neurocritical Care	
	Staff RN Stroke Unit/ Neurological Floor	
	Therapists:	
	• Physical therapy	
	• Occupational therapy	
	• Speech and language therapy	
	eICU and telemedicine	
	Radiology neuroimaging	
	Interventional neuroradiology:	
	• Coil embolization	
	• Angioplasty (mechanical or chemical)	
	• Clot extraction (MERCI or Penumbra devices)	
	• Intra-arterial lytic	
	• Intracranial and extracranial stent placement	
	Surgery:	
	• Cranial	
	• Spine	
	• Endarterectomy	
	Unit and assistant nurse managers	
	Outcomes managers, case managers, unit clerks, and social workers	
	Nurse educators	
	APN meeting	
	Office time neurology	
	Office time – neurosurgery	
	Radiation oncology	
	Hospitalist physicians	

(continued on next page)

Orientation Components	Orientation Content	Date Completed
	Rapid response team	
	Daily operations report	
	Collaboration with other NPs and PAs	
Clinical Management		
	Brain tumor:	
	• Glioblastoma multiform	
	• Astrocytoma	
	• Meningioma	
	Intracranial hemorrhage:	
	• ICH Score	
	• Blood pressure parameters for patients with or without increased intracranial pressure.	
	• Non-surgical management	
	• Surgical evacuation	
	Intraventricular hemorrhage:	
	• Assessment and management of intraventricular thrombolysis	
	Subarachnoid hemorrhage	
	Subdural hematoma	
	Decompressive craniotomy:	
	• Malignant MCA infarction	
	• Cerebellar infarction	
	• Chiari malformations	
	Pituitary tumor	
	Pneumocephalus	
	Vertebral surgeries:	
	• Anterior cervical disectomy	
	• Posterior cervical disectomy	
	• Lumbar laminectomy	
	• Management of cervical and lumbar fusions	
	Spinal cord tumor	
	Cerebral spinal fluid leak	
	Pseudomenigocele	
	Cauda equine	
	Central nervous system infections	
	History & physical	
	Preprinted orders:	
	• Neurocritical Care	
	• Hemorrhagic stroke	
	• Subarachnoid hemorrhage	
	• Electrolyte	
	• Glucose	
	• Agitation	
	• Withdrawal/Embrace hope	
	• Loop	
	• Brain death checklist	
	• Lumbar drain	

(continued on next page)

Orientation Components	Orientation Content	Date Completed
	Discharge orders:	
	• Spine	
	• Brain	
	• Skilled Nursing Facility	
	• Inpatient rehab	
	• Select	
	• Home health	
	Medication reconciliation	
	Cranial nerve exam	
	Lumbar exam	
	Cervical exam	
	Spinal cord injury:	
	• Exam	
	• Surgical stabilization	
	• Medical management	
	Fluid imbalance syndromes:	
	• Diabetes insipidis	
	• Syndrome of inappropriate antidiuretic hormone	
	• Cerebral salt wasting	
	Shunt reprogramming:	
	• Fluoroscopy	
	• Bedside	
	Ventriculostomy:	
	• Insertion	
	• Management	
	• Troubleshooting	
	• Irrigation	
	• Medication instillation	
	• Culturing	
	Lumbar Drain:	
	• Management	
	• Troubleshooting	
	• Irrigation	
	• Culturing	
	Subdural drain	
	Subgaleal drain	
	Lumbar drain:	
	• Insertion	
	• Removal	
	Intraparenchymal bolt	
	Shunts:	
	• Insertion	
	• Assessment	
	• Tap	
	Minor suturing	

(continued on next page)

Orientation Components	Orientation Content	Date Completed
	Transcranial Doppler:	
	• Vasospasm monitoring	
	• Detection of vascular occlusions	
	• Sonothrombolysis	
	• Vasomotor reactivity testing	
	• Cerebral circulatory arrest	
	• Intracranial compliance / flow resistance detection	
	Ischemic Stroke:	
	• Clinical localization by neurovascular territory	
	• NIH Stroke Scale certification	
	• Periprocedural management of intravenous thrombolysis with tPA	
	• Intra-arterial rescue – patient selection and periprocedural management	
	Neuroimaging Interpretation:	
	• Multi-modal computed tomography	
	• Multi-modal magnetic resonance imaging	
	• Digital subtraction angiography	
	• Transcranial Doppler and extracranial duplex	
	Critical Care Specific:	
	• Arterial line insertion	
	• Intubation	
	• Ventilator management and weaning	
	• Central line insertion	
	• Hemodynamic monitoring	

APPENDIX 2: ORIENTATION COMPETENCY ASSESSMENT FORM

Orientation Competency Assessment Form

Nursing Position: <u>Nurse Practitioner/Physician Assistant/Advanced Practice Nurse</u>   **Department/Unit:** <u>ICU</u>

Orientation Period: From _____ **To** _____

Associate's Name: _____ **Associate. ID #:** _____   **Director/VP:** _____

Primary/Lead Preceptors name: _____

DIRECTIONS:

PreAssess: The associate will complete the pre-assessment section form at the beginning of the orientation to indicate her/his level of experience using the following
codes: **NE** = No experience   **LE** = Limited Experience   **NR** = Needs review/ Needs to review the policy
C = Can perform independently   **P** = Proficient (Can teach others & perform independently)

Competency Assessment: To be utilized by the preceptor/educator
1. For each competency, please circle either: **Y** = Met **N** = Not met, or **N/A** = not applicable
2. Initial and Date the evaluator column when the competency is validated.
3. ***Provide evaluation/action plan for any competency rated "N"****

Methods of validation are abbreviated as follows: **D** = Demonstration   **R** = Hospital Records   **S** = Simulation   **T** = Written Test   **V** = Verbalized Correct Steps
Action plan abbreviations: **OD**= Observe & Repeat Demonstration   **PR**= Policy/Procedure Review   **RT**= Retake Test/Case Study   **AI**= Attend Inservice/Class
WP= Work Practice observation

Reference abbreviations: **SOC**= standard of care **P&P**= Policy and Procedure **Adm** = Administrative Policy Manual,
NU = Nursing Policy manual, **Safety** = Safety manual **SLM**= self-learning module   **PC**= Performance Criteria
PBDS=Performance Based Development System

1/04

General Hospital

SELF PRE-ASSESS	COMPETENCY	MET (Y=Met, N=Not met, N/A=Not applicable)	METHOD	REFERENCE	EVALUATOR & DATE	EVALUATION/ACTION PLAN (If Applicable)
NE LE P NR C	**Communication:** demonstrates ability to correctly follow established standards • Follows chain of command in reporting variances	Y N	D	Hospital Specific Phone systems, call light system		
NE LE P NR C	**Confidentiality/Patient Rights:** maintains according to policy	Y N	D	P & P		
NE LE P NR C	**Advance Directives/Code Status**	Y N	D	P & P		
NE LE P NR C	**Computer Skills:** demonstrates ability to use computer for basic functions related to job description	Y N	D,S	Hospital Specific		
NE LE P NR C	**Customer Satisfaction:** meets established expectation	Y N	D	Customer Service Training		
NE LE P NR C	**Cultural Diversity:** Demonstrates cultural awareness and skill in delivering care to diverse patient populations	Y N	D	Resources for Cultural Diversity www.ethnomed.org www.diversityrx.org		
NE LE P NR C	**Documentation:** provides accurate and timely documentation appropriate to department and position. • Performs patient/family education utilizing the resources available and documents appropriately.	Y N	D	P&P SOC Hospital Specific Addendum		
NE LE P NR C	**Environment of Care:** performs consistently within established standards • Demonstrates appropriate response to clinical alarms and assures alarms functional • Demonstrates appropriate response to emergency codes: fire, weather, disaster, infant abduction, cardiopulmonary arrest	Y N	D	SOC P&P Infection Control/Safety Manual BLS Disaster Manual		
NE LE P NR C	**Body Mechanics:** utilizes appropriate safety equipment	Y N	D	P&P Unit specific equipment addendum		
NE LE P NR C	**Performance Improvement:** verbalizes knowledge of organizational initiatives and unit/hospital based projects	Y N	V	P&P SOC		

SELF PRE-ASSESS	COMPETENCY	MET	METHOD	REFERENCE	EVAL-UATOR & DATE	EVALUATION/ACTION PLAN (If Applicable)
NE LE P / NR C	Age related care: provides appropriate to age of the patient	Y	D	SOC		
NE LE P / NR C	Values: demonstrates conduct that supports	Y	D	St. John Health Values		
NE LE P / NR C	Corporate and Regulatory Compliance: verbalizes role in	Y	D,T	HIPPA, Corp Compliance Training Corporate Checklist		
NE LE P / NR C	Patient Identification: practices according to policy	Y	D	P & P		

SELF PRE-ASSESS	COMPETENCY	MET Y=Met N=Not met N/A=Not applicable	METHOD	REFERENCE	EVAL-UATOR & DATE	EVALUATION/ACTION PLAN (If Applicable)
	General Unit					
NE LE P / NR C	Patient Abuse: explains age appropriate reporting and documenting procedures according to policy/procedure	Y N	D	P&P		
NE LE P / NR C	Equipment: Utilizes equipment safely according to orientation and unit specific equipment addendum.	Y N	D,S	P&P Unit specific equipment addendum		
NE LE P / NR C	Patient Assessment: demonstrates ability to perform a complete history and physical to diagnose, prescribe and treat health responses for individual patients. • Develops, implements and evaluates complex intervention strategies, revises plan to reflect dynamic needs of the patient • Orders and interprets diagnostic tests, orders diet, patient activity, and medication therapy. • Orders consultations with other disciplines and specialties in collaboration with the Intensivist	Y N	D	SOC		

NE	LE	NR	C	P		Y	N		
					Daily Care/Complex Care Rounds: provides comprehensive clinical coordination for assigned patient group • Initiates referrals to appropriate health care providers within the healthcare system • Coordinates discharge planning in collaboration with the multidisciplinary team • Evaluates and documents patient response to intervention, rounds with attending physician. • Documents admission, pre-op, transfer and daily progress notes	Y	N	D	P&P SOC
					Continuous Quality Assurance: • **Keystone ICU**	Y	N	D, PR	P & P SOC
					Delegation: assigns appropriate responsibilities to unlicensed assistive /licensed personnel • May give verbal or telephone orders to the staff nurses and other disciplines	Y	N	D	SOC P&P **Hospital Plan for the Provision of Patient Care**
					Emergency Care: participates in emergency situations including: • RRT • Codes/Stats • Unit specific patient placement guidelines	Y	N	D,S	SOC P&P **Hospital Plan for the Provision of Patient Care**
					Lab Draws: performs lab draws according to policy • **Phlebotomy:** Performs peripheral lab draws according to policy • **Central Lines:** Performs central line lab draws according to policy	Y	N	D, S	SOC P&P

				Y	N	D	SOC P&P
NE	NR	LE	C	P	**Medication**		
					Administration/Reconciliation: administers medications safely via		
					• PO		
					• IM		
					• SQ		
					• IVPB		
					• IVP		
					• N/G		
					• Feeding tube		
					• Transdermal routes		
					• Use of Pyxis System		
					• Reconciles medications at admission, transfer and discharge		
					• Tight Glycemic Control		
NE	NR	LE	C	P	**Alcohol Withdrawal Protocol:** assesses patient for and performs according to policy	Y	N	D	SOC P&P
NE	NR	LE	C	P	**Restraints: assesses patient, orders and documents per policy**	Y	N	D	SOC P&P
NE	NR	LE	C	P	**Assesses need for patient safety sitter**	Y	N	D	SOC P&P
NE	NR	LE	C	P	**Admissions, Transfers, Discharges and Patient Handoff:** carries out according to policy	Y	N	D	SOC P&P
NE	NR	LE	C	P	**Pain Management:** assesses and prescribes appropriate pain management plan in collaboration with Intensivist	Y	N	D	SOC, P&P
NE	NR	LE	C	P	**Skin Care:** Assesses and prescribes appropriate therapy for potential and actual skin breakdown.	Y	N	D	SOC P&P
					• Performs minor debridment and packing		
					• Orders specialty beds as appropriate		

SELF PRE-ASSESS	COMPETENCY	Y	N	D	REFERENCE		COMMENTS/ACTION PLAN
NE LE P NR C	**Expiration Care:** Identifies appropriate procedure when patient expires. • Coroners Cases • Autopsy Procedure • Body Disposition Form				SOC P&P		

SELF PRE-ASSESS	COMPETENCY	MET Y=Met N=Not met N/A= Not applicable	METHOD	REFERENCE	EVAL-UATOR & DATE	COMMENTS/ACTION PLAN (If Applicable)
	Department Specific: ***Critical Care/ICU*** Organizing Frameworks: Body Systems and Patient Populations					
NE LE P NR C	**Care of the patient with** **Cardiovascular Dysfunction** • Cardiovascular assessment	Y N	D, R, S T, V	SOC Clinical Guidelines		
NE LE P NR C	• Care of the patient with Heart Failure- Pathway	Y N	D, R, S T, V	SOC Clinical Guidelines		
	• Care of the patient with Acute Myocardial Infarction-Pathway	Y N	D, R, S T, V	SOC Clinical Guidelines		
	• Care of the patient post cardiac catheterization	Y N	D, R, S T, V	SOC P&P		
	• Care of the patient post cardiac catheterization intervention	Y N	D, R, S T, V	SOC P&P		
	Cardiac Emergencies: demonstrates **ability to correctly follow established** **policies for:**					
NE LE P NR C	• Defibrillation/Monitor	Y N	D, R, S T, V	P & P		
NE LE P NR C	• Cardioversion	Y N	D, R, S T, V	P& P		
NE LE P NR C	• Automated External Defibrillation	Y N	D, R, S T, V	P & P		

Care of the Patient with a Cardiac Pacemakers: manages					
• Temporary transvenous and epicardial pacing	NE LE P / NR C	Y	N	D, R, S / T, V	P&P
• Permanent pacemaker (assessing function)/ICD	NE LE P / NR C	Y	N	D, R, S / T, V	SOC / P&P
• Temporary transcutaneous (external)pacing	NE LE P / NR C	Y	N	D, R, S / T, V	P&P
Care of the patient with electrocardiographic monitoring; provides care and demonstrates correct usage					
• Hardwire and telemetry	NE LE P / NR C	Y	N	D, R, S / T, V	P&P
• EKG/Rhythm Interpretation	NE LE P / NR C	Y	N	D, R, S / T, V	P&P / SOC
• Demonstrates appropriate method of individualizing alarm parameters based on patient need.	NE LE P / NR C	Y	N	D, R, S / T, V	Performance Criterion Checklist / P&P
Care of the patient with central venous access and invasive hemodynamic monitoring: manages					
• Arterial Catheter Insertion (assist), Care and Removal	NE LE P / NR C	Y	N	D, R, S / T, V	P&P / SOC
Central/Venous Lines: assesses need for and care of: • PICC lines • Implanted ports: accessing • Single and multiple lumen catheters	NE LE P / NR C	Y	N	D, R, S / T, V	
Arterial and Venous Sheath Removal: performs	NE LE P / NR C	Y	N	V, D x 3	P&P
Care of the patient receiving vasoactive and antidysrhythmic IV medications:	NE LE P / NR C	Y	N	D, R, S / T, V	P & P / SOC
• Calculates doses, flow rates and administration of continuous intravenous infusions					

Care of the patient with Pulmonary Dysfunction

	NE LE P / NR C		Y	N			
•	Ongoing pulmonary assessment		Y	N	D, R, S T, V	SOC	
•	Care of the patient with COPD/Asthma		Y	N	D, R, S T, V	SOC Clinical Guideline	
•	Care of the patient with Pneumonia		Y	N	D, R, S T, V	SOC Clinical Guideline	
•	O2 monitoring by pulse oximetry		Y	N	D, R, S T, V	SOC	
•	ABG Interpretation		Y	N	D, R, S T, V	SOC	
•	Incentive Spirometry		Y	N	D, R, S T, V	SOC	
•	Endotracheal intubation and extubation		Y	N	D, R, S T, V	SOC P&P	
•	Oral and nasopharyngeal airway insertion		Y	N	D, R, S T, V	SOC P&P	
•	O2 adjuncts setup and delivery		Y	N	D, R, S T, V	SOC P&P	
•	Endotracheal and Tracheostomy tube suctioning		Y	N	D, R, S T, V	SOC P&P	
•	Nasal tracheal suctioning		Y	N	D, R, S T, V	SOC P&P	
•	Tracheostomy care		Y	N	D, R, S T, V	SOC P&P	
•	Assist with chest tube insertion and removal		Y	N	D, R, S T, V	SOC P&P	
•	Closed chest drainage system		Y	N	D, R, S T, V	SOC P&P	

Care of the patient on a ventilator: manages						
NE LE P / NR C	• Ventilatory management–volume and pressure modes	Y	N	D, R, S T, V		SOC
NE LE P / NR C	• Standard weaning criteria (NIF, PEEP, TV, VC	Y	N	D, R, S T, V		SOC
NE LE P / NR C	• Weaning Procedure	Y	N	D, R, S T, V		SOC
Care of the patient with Neurological dysfunction						
NE LE P / NR C	• Neurological Assessment	Y	N	D, R, S T, V		SOC
NE LE P / NR C	• Care of the patient with Acute Brain Attack	Y	N	D, R, S T, V		SOC Clinical Guideline
Care of the patient with gastrointestinal system dysfunction: provides management of:						
NE LE P / NR C	• Gastrointestinal assessment	Y	N	D, R, S T, V		SOC
NE LE P / NR C	• Care of the patient with GI Bleed	Y	N	D, R, S T, V		SOC Clinical Guideline
NE LE P / NR C	• Gastric lavage in hemorrhage and overdose	Y	N	D, R, S T, V		SOC P&P
NE LE P / NR C	• Orogastric and nasogastric tube insertion, care and removal	Y	N	D, R, S T, V		SOC P&P
NE LE P / NR C	• Care of the patient with PEG or Jejunostomy tube	Y	N	D, R, S T, V		SOC P&P
NE LE P / NR C	• Small bore feeding tube insertion	Y	N	D, R, S T, V		SOC P&P
Care of the patient with genitourinary system dysfunction: provides management of:						
NE LE P / NR C	• Genitourinary assessment: including bladderscan	Y	N	D, R, S T, V		SOC P&P
NE LE P / NR C	• Foley catheter insertion, care, removal	Y	N	D, R, S T, V		SOC P&P

NE	LE	P	• Genitourinary catheter irrigation: intermittent and continuous	Y	N	D, R, S T, V		SOC P&P			
NR	C										
NE	LE	P	• Care of patient with: urinary stent, nephrostomy tubes, urostomy	Y	N	D, R, S T, V		SOC P&P			
NR	C										
			Care of the patient with renal system dysfunction: manages								
NE	LE	P	• Care of the patient with dialysis access device: fistula, shunt, hemodialysis catheter	Y	N	D, R, S T, V		SOC P&P			
NR	C										
NE	LE	P	• Hemodialysis (Assist)	Y	N	D, R, S T, V		SOC P&P			
NR	C										
NE	LE	P	• Peritoneal Dialysis	Y	N	D, R, S T, V		SOC P&P			
NR	C										
NE	LE	P	**Care of the surgical patient** • Pre-op care • Post op care • Care of the patient undergoing bowel surgery	Y	N	D, R, S T, V		SOC P&P Clinical Guidelines			
NR	C										
NE	LE	P	**Care of the patient with endocrine dysfunction: DKA/HHNK** • Demonstrates appropriate use of insulin protocols	Y	N	D, R, S T, V		SOC P&P Clinical Guidelines			
NR	C										
NE	LE	P	**Wound Care: care of the patient with wounds including** • Wound Vac • Simple & Complex Dressing Changes	Y	N	D, R, S T, V		SOC P&P			
NR	C										
NE	LE	P	**Care of the patient with End of Life issues** • Palliative Care • Hospice Care • Ethics Committee (Role of/Accessing)	Y	N	D, R, S T, V		P&P SOC			
NR	C										

				Y	N	D, R, S T, V	P&P
NE	LE	P	• Identification of potential organ donors: Gift of Life	Y	N	D, R, S T, V	P&P
NR	C						
NE	LE	P	• Care of the organ donor	Y	N	D, R, S T, V	P&P
NR	C						
NE	LE	P	• Request for organ donation	Y	N	D, R, S T, V	P&P
NR	C						
NE	LE	P	• Withdrawing life sustaining support	Y	N	D, R, S T, V	P&P
NR	C						
NE	LE	P	• Psychosocial support	Y	N	D, R, S T, V	SOC
NR	C						

Care of the Patient with Sepsis

NE	LE	P	• Identification of patients with SIRS/sepsis	Y			
NR	C			N			
			• Demonstrates use of sepsis bundle				

Preceptor Signatures: _____

Orientation Competencies Completed: _____   Associate Signature: _____

Final Review Date: _____

VP Signature: _____

Action Plan for those items "Not Met":

Erratum

An error occurred in the article "Creating a Culture of Change Through Implementation of a Safe Patient Handling Program" by Karen Stenger, Volume 19, Issue 2, Page 220 (June 2007). An inaccuracy was discovered in the data table on page 220 and in the data referring to that table.

We apologize for this oversight.

Data in Table 1 should read

Annual Report	2002	2003	2004
Total IOSH recordable cases	51	76	67
Total IOSH days lost	695	608	404
Total workers comp cost	$698,111	$303,669	$74,125
Workers comp cost reduction from 2002		57%	89%

The analysis in the article (page 220) is inaccurate based on this new knowledge. Incorporating what was recently discovered, this should have read, beginning in the second paragraph after (Table 1) reference:

"From 2002–2004, lost work days decreased from 695 to 404, a 42% reduction. If UIHC replaced every one of the 291 lost workdays with another employee, it would be equivalent to hiring another full time employee. The cost estimate for one RN full time employee, salaried conservatively, including benefits, would be approximately $66,000. From 2002 to 2004, worker's compensation cost fell from $698,111 to $74,125, indicating an 89% reduction. In 3 years, UIHC reduced workers' compensation costs by more than $620,000. UIHC saw an increase in the number of OSHA recordable patient exertions. From 2002 to 2004, recordable exertions increased 31% from 51 to 67."

This portion refers to the abstract that appears in the table of contents and online:

"Health care professionals have a high risk for being injured while moving patients manually. The University of Iowa Hospitals and Clinics (UIHC) realized a need to reduce injuries suffered during patient movement. A UIHC multidisciplinary task force consulted the latest research, trialed products, and involved employees in selecting equipment for and implementing a safe patient handling program. This program resulted in a 42% reduction in lost workdays and an 89% reduction in workers' compensation costs. The keys to this program were involving employees, partnering with a key vendor, engaging change agents at the unit level, and applying persistence and re-education to staff."

Crit Care Nurs Clin N Am 21 (2009) 595
doi:10.1016/j.ccell.2009.09.002
0899-5885/09/$ – see front matter © 2009 Elsevier Inc. All rights reserved.

ccnursing.theclinics.com

Index

Note: Page numbers of article titles are in **boldface** type.

Crit Care Nurs Clin N Am 21 (2009) 597–604
doi:10.1016/S0899-5885(09)00107-5
0899-5885/09/$ – see front matter © 2009 Elsevier Inc. All rights reserved.

ccnursing.theclinics.com

United States Postal Service

Statement of Ownership, Management, and Circulation
(All Periodicals Publications Except Requestor Publications)

1. Publication Title	2. Publication Number								3. Filing Date
Critical Care Nursing Clinics of North America	0	0	6	-	2	7	7	3	9/15/09

4. Issue Frequency	5. Number of Issues Published Annually	6. Annual Subscription Price
Mar, Jun, Sep, Dec	4	$130.00

7. Complete Mailing Address of Known Office of Publication (Not printer) (Street, city, county, state, and ZIP+4®)

Elsevier Inc.
360 Park Avenue South
New York, NY 10010-1710

Contact Person
Stephen Bushing
Telephone (Include area code)
215-239-3688

8. Complete Mailing Address of Headquarters or General Business Office of Publisher (Not printer)

Elsevier Inc., 360 Park Avenue South, New York, NY 10010-1710

9. Full Names and Complete Mailing Addresses of Publisher, Editor, and Managing Editor (Do not leave blank)

Publisher (Name and complete mailing address)

John Schrefer, Elsevier, Inc., 1600 John F. Kennedy Blvd. Suite 1800, Philadelphia, PA 19103-2899

Editor (Name and complete mailing address)

Katie Hartner, Elsevier, Inc., 1600 John F. Kennedy Blvd. Suite 1800, Philadelphia, PA 19103-2899

Managing Editor (Name and complete mailing address)

Catherine Bewick, Elsevier, Inc., 1600 John F. Kennedy Blvd. Suite 1800, Philadelphia, PA 19103-2899

10. Owner (Do not leave blank. If the publication is owned by a corporation, give the name and address of the corporation immediately followed by the names and addresses of all stockholders owning or holding 1 percent or more of the total amount of stock. If not owned by a corporation, give the names and addresses of the individual owners. If owned by a partnership or other unincorporated firm, give its name and address as well as those of each individual owner. If the publication is published by a nonprofit organization, give its name and address.)

Full Name	Complete Mailing Address
Wholly owned subsidiary of	4520 East-West Highway
Reed/Elsevier, US holdings	Bethesda, MD 20814

11. Known Bondholders, Mortgagees, and Other Security Holders Owning or Holding 1 Percent or More of Total Amount of Bonds, Mortgages, or Other Securities. If none, check box. ☐ None

Full Name	Complete Mailing Address
N/A	

12. Tax Status (For completion by nonprofit organizations authorized to mail at nonprofit rates) (Check one)
The purpose, function, and nonprofit status of this organization and the exempt status for federal income tax purposes:
☐ Has Not Changed During Preceding 12 Months
☐ Has Changed During Preceding 12 Months (Publisher must submit explanation of change with this statement)

PS Form 3526, September 2007 (Page 1 of 3 (Instructions Page 3)) PSN 7530-01-000-9931 PRIVACY NOTICE: See our Privacy policy in www.usps.com

13. Publication Title			14. Issue Date for Circulation Data Below
Critical Care Nursing Clinics of North America			June 2009

15. Extent and Nature of Circulation		Average No. Copies Each Issue During Preceding 12 Months	No. Copies of Single Issue Published Nearest to Filing Date
a. Total Number of Copies (Net press run)		1325	1100
b. Paid Circulation (By Mail and Outside the Mail)	(1) Mailed Outside-County Paid Subscriptions Stated on PS Form 3541. (Include paid distribution above nominal rate, advertiser's proof copies, and exchange copies)	698	619
	(2) Mailed In-County Paid Subscriptions Stated on PS Form 3541 (Include paid distribution above nominal rate, advertiser's proof copies, and exchange copies)		
	(3) Paid Distribution Outside the Mails Including Sales Through Dealers and Carriers, Street Vendors, Counter Sales, and Other Paid Distribution Outside USPS®	144	129
	(4) Paid Distribution by Other Classes Mailed Through the USPS (e.g. First-Class Mail®)		
c. Total Paid Distribution (Sum of 15b (1), (2), (3), and (4))		842	748
d. Free or Nominal Rate Distribution (By Mail and Outside the Mail)	(1) Free or Nominal Rate Outside-County Copies Included on PS Form 3541	77	80
	(2) Free or Nominal Rate In-County Copies Included on PS Form 3541		
	(3) Free or Nominal Rate Copies Mailed at Other Classes Through the USPS (e.g. First-Class Mail)		
	(4) Free or Nominal Rate Distribution Outside the Mail (Carriers or other means)		
e. Total Free or Nominal Rate Distribution (Sum of 15d (1), (2), (3) and (4))		77	80
f. Total Distribution (Sum of 15c and 15e)		919	828
g. Copies not Distributed (See instructions to publishers #4 (page #3))		406	272
h. Total (Sum of 15f and g)		1325	1100
i. Percent Paid (15c divided by 15f times 100)		91.62%	90.34%

16. Publication of Statement of Ownership

☐ If the publication is a general publication, publication of this statement is required. Will be printed in the December 2009 issue of this publication. ☐ Publication not required

17. Signature and Title of Editor, Publisher, Business Manager, or Owner

Stephen R. Bushing – Subscription Services Coordinator

Date September 15, 2009

I certify that all information furnished on this form is true and complete. I understand that anyone who furnishes false or misleading information on this form or who omits material or information requested on the form may be subject to criminal sanctions (including fines and imprisonment) and/or civil sanctions (including civil penalties).

PS Form 3526, September 2007 (Page 2 of 3)

Moving?

Make sure your subscription moves with you!

To notify us of your new address, find your **Clinics Account Number** (located on your mailing label above your name), and contact customer service at:

Email: journalscustomerservice-usa@elsevier.com

800-654-2452 (subscribers in the U.S. & Canada)
314-447-8871 (subscribers outside of the U.S. & Canada)

Fax number: 314-447-8029

Elsevier Health Sciences Division
Subscription Customer Service
3251 Riverport Lane
Maryland Heights, MO 63043

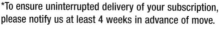
*To ensure uninterrupted delivery of your subscription, please notify us at least 4 weeks in advance of move.